Echocardiography

in primary care

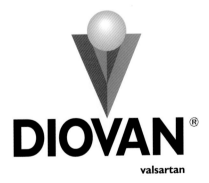

DIOVAN®

valsartan

Echocardiography

in primary care

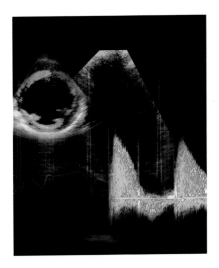

John Chambers MA, MD, FRCP

Senior Lecturer and Consultant in Cardiology
Guy's Hospital, London, UK

The Parthenon Publishing Group

International Publishers in Medicine, Science & Technology

NEW YORK   LONDON

Published in the USA by
The Parthenon Publishing Group Inc.
One Blue Hill Plaza, PO Box 1564
Pearl River, New York 10965, USA

Published in the UK by
The Parthenon Publishing Group Limited
Casterton Hall, Carnforth
Lancs LA6 2LA, UK

ISBN 1-85070-909-2

Design and artwork: Rowland & Hird, Lancaster
Printed and bound by T. G. Hostench S. A., Spain

Contents

Dedication

This book is dedicated to Dr John Wells.

John Wells qualified as a doctor from University College, London in 1930. After completing hospital posts in Norwich and Nottingham, he worked as a general practitioner on the Isles of Scilly from 1936 to 1945. During this period he collaborated with established artists living in St. Ives, Cornwall including Ben Nicholson, Barbara Hepworth and Naum Gabbo. After the Second World War he moved to Newlyn in Cornwall to work full-time as a painter. Many of his abstract images take inspiration from organic subjects like the line of a shore or the flight of a bird. John Wells transforms observations founded in a scientific methodology with the genius of an artist. Conversely, through the artistic beauty of an image, he allows us to glimpse the pure beauty of physics. This is all too small a tribute to a great artist at the approach of his 90th birthday.

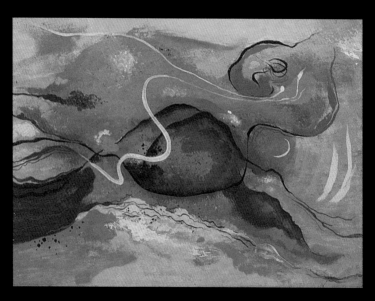

Isles of Scilly, Cornwall, 1944. This image was painted whilst
Dr John Wells was a general practitioner on Scilly

Preface

Most textbooks of echocardiography are systematic treatments from a mainly technical standpoint. The use of echocardiography, however, has long ago expanded beyond the boundaries of the specialised cardiac unit. General physicians, general practitioners and primary care physicians now request an increasing proportion of studies and need to know what clinical questions modern echocardiography can answer. This short book presents echocardiography from the general clinical perspective.

Acknowledgements

I wish to thank Helen Rimington who collated most of the data in Chapter 2. I should also like to thank Philip Cummin and George Adam for their comments on the manuscript. Many colleagues in general practice have helped indirectly with discussions about the place of echocardiography in general practice and these include George Adam, Lesley Chambers, Philip Cummin, Paul Hobday, Caroline Jessel, Paul Lewis, Nigel Minett and Martin Moss. Once again, thanks to Helen Kennett who graciously loaned me for putting together this book. Some of the illustrations have appeared in *Clinical Echocardiography* by John Chambers published by BMJ books.

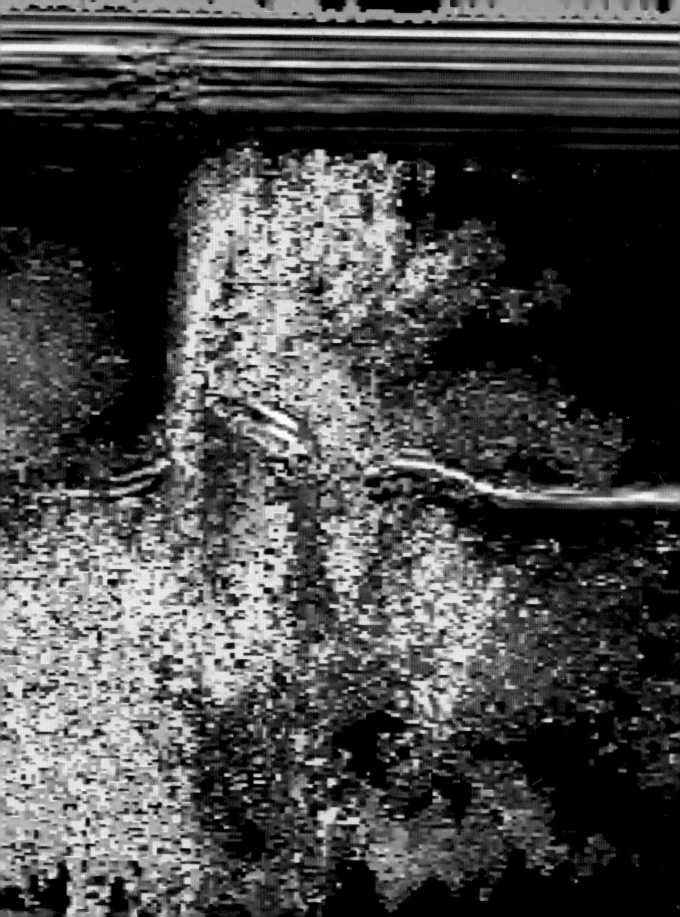

Summary of indications for open-access echocardiography

- Suspected heart failure

  Unexplained breathlessness
  Clinical signs of heart failure but aetiology uncertain

- Murmur

  A diastolic murmur or a pansystolic or long ejection systolic murmur or any murmur associated with cardiac symptoms

- Borderline hypertension

- Atrial fibrillation

- Screening

  First-degree relatives of patients with hypertrophic cardiomyopathy
  Possible collagen abnormalities e.g. Marfan syndrome

Echocardiography is not indicated in most patients with:

- Syncope or dizzy spells

- A short soft ejection systolic murmur with a normal second heart sound and no symptoms

- A minor increase in cardiothoracic ratio on the chest radiograph without breathlessness

- Atypical chest pain

- Transient ischaemic attack or stroke with a normal electrocardiogram and cardiovascular examination.

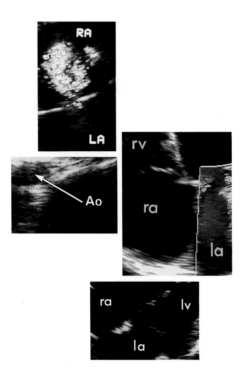

Key to figure abbreviations

LA left atrium
LV left ventricle
RV right ventricle
RA right atrium
P pericardium
PW posterior wall
S septum
Ao aorta
RCA right coronary artery
LAD left anterior descending
PA pulmonary artery
Cx circumflex
ASD atrial septal defect
VSD ventricular septal defect

Chapter 1

Echocardiographic techniques

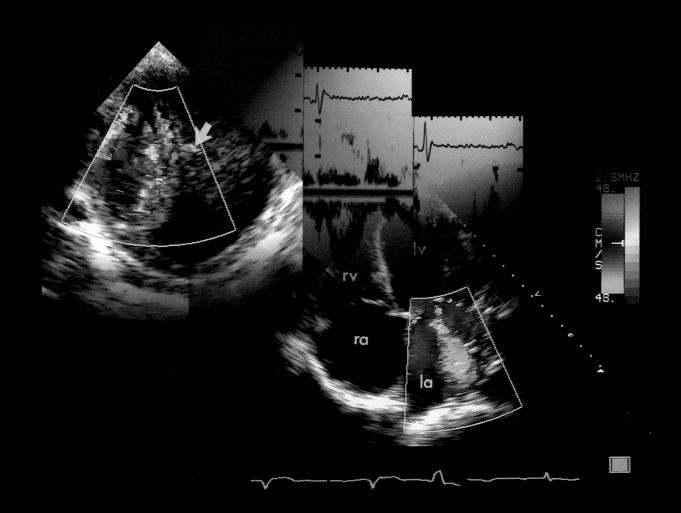

Echocardiography provides information about the anatomy and physiology of the heart. It can detect and quantify the severity of most congenital or acquired heart disorders, and may suggest an aetiology. Echocardiography includes both imaging (two-dimensional, and M-mode), and Doppler modalities (continuous wave, pulsed, and colour flow mapping). These all rely on the piezoelectric effect in which a crystal is made to vibrate by the passage of an electric current. This generates ultrasound waves which are transmitted into the body with a small proportion being reflected back. The modalities, which can be used separately or together (Table 1.1), differ most in the way that the reflected ultrasound is collected and analysed.

Two-dimensional echocardiography

Most of a transmitted pulse of ultrasound is scattered or absorbed, but a little is reflected at interfaces between tissues of different density, for example between right ventricular blood and septal endocardium (Figure 1.1, arrow). Reflected ultrasound distorts the piezoelectric crystal and produces an electric current, the size of which controls the density of a spot on the display screen. The position of this spot is determined by the time difference between transmission and return of the ultrasound. After allowing enough time to collect reflected ultrasound from the deepest parts of the heart, a further pulse is transmitted along the next scan line.

Table 1.1 Modalities of echocardiography and their uses

Modality	Principal uses
Two-dimensional imaging	Anatomy Valve and ventricular motion
M-mode	Timing of events Dimensions
Colour flow mapping	Detection of regurgitation or shunts Semiquantitative assessment of regurgitation
Continuous wave Doppler	Estimation of severity of valve stenosis and regurgitation
Pulsed Doppler	Calculation of stroke volume Left ventricular diastolic function Effective orifice area in aortic stenosis

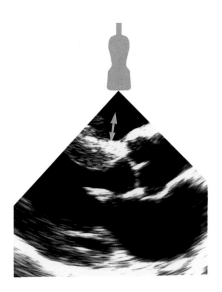

Fig 1.1 Two-dimensional echocardiogram illustrating reflection of ultrasound from the right ventricular cavity/endocardial interface. The transducer position is always at the apex of the image (as illustrated)

To form a typical image using conventional technology, pulses are transmitted along scan lines (about 120 over a 90° arc) at least 20–30 times a second. The ultrasound beam moves either by rotation of a mechanical head, or by electronic steering. Substantial processing is carried out within the equipment to compensate for problems such as attenuation of the signal, or divergence of the scan lines.

Two-dimensional echocardiography is used for detecting abnormal anatomy or movement. It can also be used to measure cavity dimensions if M-mode is technically impossible or if areas or volumes are required (e.g. mitral valve orifice area or left ventricular end-systolic volume).

M-mode echocardiography

M-mode stands for motion mode. An M-mode recording (Figure 1.2) is constructed by transmitting and receiving ultrasound

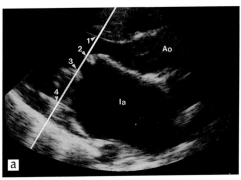

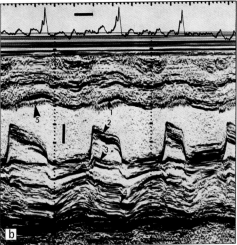

Fig 1.2 M-mode and two-dimensional echocardiograms in a patient with rheumatic mitral stenosis. An M-mode scan line has been chosen through the tips of the mitral leaflets. The following structures may be seen on both the two-dimensional (**a**) and M-mode image (**b**): left septal echo (**1**); tip of anterior mitral leaflet (**2**); posterior leaflet (**3**); posterior left ventricular wall (**4**). There is also vibration of the left septal echo as a result of coexistent aortic regurgitation (**5**). In the M-mode image, the vertical bar represents 1 cm and the horizontal bar 200 ms

along only one scan line, thus giving substantially greater sensitivity than two-dimensional echocardiography for recording moving structures. The returning echoes are displayed as a graph of depth against time.

M-mode is used for timing events within the heart and measurement of cardiac dimensions. It should only be applied if the cursor can be aligned perpendicular to the structure being assessed.

Continuous wave Doppler

In the main Doppler modalities ultrasound is reflected from moving red blood cells. The Doppler principle is then used to derive velocity information from the frequency shift that occurs between transmitted and reflected ultrasound. The frequency shift (Δf) is twice the transmitting frequency ($2.f_0$) multiplied by the blood velocity corrected for angle ($v.\cos\theta$) and divided by the speed of sound (c). This is the same principle as the sound of a car horn rising in pitch as the car approaches and falling as it recedes. If red blood cells are moving towards the transducer when they reflect ultrasound, the reflected wavelength will be contracted; if they are moving away, the wavelength will be drawn out. Computerised analysis of the returning Doppler signal allows velocity and direction to be encoded. By convention,

velocities towards the transducer are displayed above the line, and away from it below the line.

A continuous wave Doppler transducer consists of two crystals, one transmitting continuously, the other receiving continuously. The Doppler frequency shift is in the audible range, and the audio signal is used to guide the transducer to obtain the best visual display. This display is a graph of velocity against time, with an additional densitometric dimension because the density of any spot is related to the number of red cells moving at that velocity. For example, in a recording from the left intercostal space with the transducer aimed towards a stenotic pulmonary valve, the display is most dense near the baseline (Figure 1.3, arrow), reflecting the fact that most of the blood above and below the valve is moving at a low velocity (about 1 m/s). Blood accelerating through the valve is at higher velocities, up to 5 m/s.

Continuous wave Doppler is used to estimate the severity of valve stenoses and pulmonary artery pressure and can give a semiquantitative assessment of regurgitation (see also Figures 4.11, 4.14). The technique can measure high velocities, but is limited by being unable to localise a flow signal, which could originate from anywhere along the length and width of the ultrasound beam.

Fig 1.3 Continuous wave recording in pulmonary stenosis, showing velocity and time on the vertical and horizontal axes, respectively. The signal has been recorded from the left parasternal position. The dense part of the signal (arrow) is mainly from blood moving within the right ventricle; the high-velocity signal is from blood passing through the stenotic valve

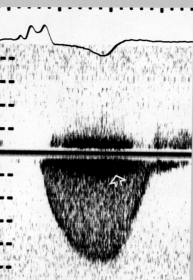

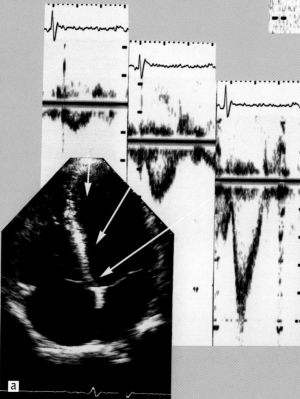

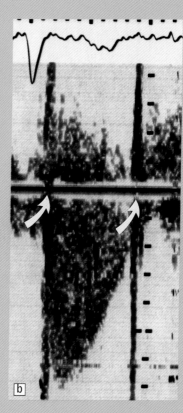

Fig 1.4 Pulsed Doppler recordings at various levels in the left ventricle between the apex and subaortic region illustrating the localising ability of pulsed Doppler (**a**). Since flow is laminar, velocities at any point vary only over a narrow range and, therefore, each waveform has a thin outline. By comparison, the continuous wave trace (**b**) records flow along the whole length of the beam. Effectively, it is the summation of all the individual pulsed waveforms that could be recorded along its length and is therefore 'filled in'. The artefacts caused by the aortic valve opening and closing are arrowed

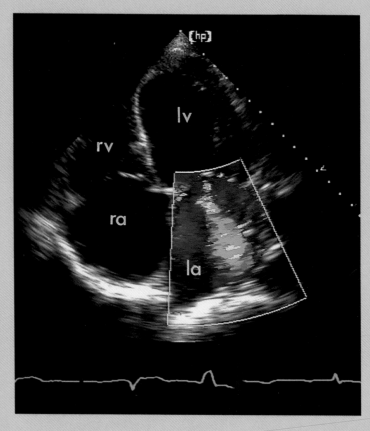

Fig 1.5 Colour flow map showing mitral regurgitation. This is an apical four-chamber view in a patient with an anterior infarct. There is a jet of mitral regurgitation within the left atrium

Fig 1.6 Aortic dissection on transoesophageal echocardiography. The flap is seen dividing true from false lumen (**a**). Colour mapping shows flow within the true lumen with a small jet (arrow) escaping through a tear into the false lumen (**b**)

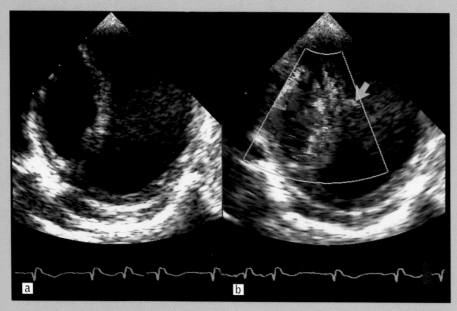

Pulsed Doppler

The need to localise a flow disturbance, or to record velocity information from a relatively small region, led to the development of pulsed Doppler. A single crystal transmits and then receives ultrasound after a preset time delay. Reflected signals are recorded only from a depth corresponding to half the product of the time delay and the speed of sound. This modality is usually combined with two-dimensional imaging in the same transducer, so that the region where velocities are measured can be localised approximately by placing a 'sample volume' over the image on the screen (Figure 2.8b). Pulsed Doppler is mainly used to describe diastolic behaviour of the left ventricle (see also Figures 2.8, 3.7), and to calculate stroke volume for use in the calculation of effective valve orifice area (Figure 4.9), cardiac output (see also Figure 3.6), and intracardiac shunts. Because the time-delay limits the rate at which a waveform can be sampled, there is a limit to the maximum velocity that can be detected accurately.

Colour flow Doppler mapping

Colour flow mapping is effectively an automated two-dimensional version of pulsed Doppler and calculates mean blood velocity and direction of flow at multiple points down alternate scan lines of an image. Using colour encoding, the velocity information is then superimposed on the image. By convention, velocities towards the transducer are displayed in red, and those away in blue. Increasing velocities are shown initially in progressively lighter shades, or changes of hue. Above a threshold velocity, a reversal of colour occurs, which aids visual detection of abnormal flow. Thus, a mitral regurgitation jet in the left atrium appears blue with some additional yellows (Figure 1.5). Often pixels where there is a wide range of velocities are depicted in green which highlights turbulence or regions of high flow acceleration.

Colour mapping is used as a screening tool for abnormal blood flow particularly for regurgitant jets or shunts. It can also give a semiquantitative estimate of the severity of regurgitation (see also Figures 4.10, 4.15).

Transoesophageal echocardiography

In echocardiography there is always a trade-off between attenuation and resolution. Lower frequency transducers, as required for most transthoracic imaging, have good penetration, but relatively poor resolution. The transoesophageal approach has the advantage that the oesophagus is separated from the base of the heart and aorta by at most 0.5 cm of tissue. This means that attenuation of ultrasound is small and a relatively high frequency

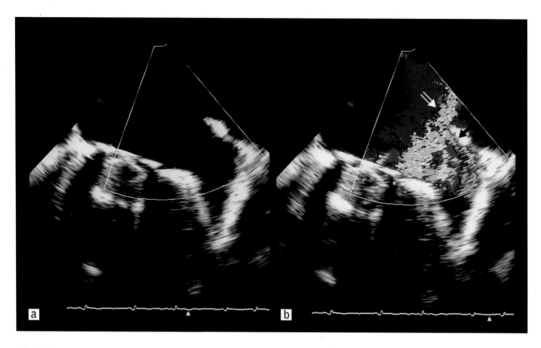

Fig 1.7 Transoesophageal echocardiogram in a patient with a mechanical prosthetic valve in the mitral position. In (**a**) there are two normal transprosthetic leaks. In (**b**) there is a large paraprosthetic jet dividing into two with one branch remaining in the left atrium (⇒) and the other entering the left atrial appendage (→)

transducer can be used, mounted on a modified gastroscope. Furthermore, structures, like the descending thoracic aorta or atria which are distant from the chest wall and therefore hard to image transthoracically, are closely adjacent to the oesophagus. A mechanical valve in the mitral position shields the left atrium which prevents ultrasound entering from the transthoracic approach, but this is not a problem *via* the 'backdoor' approach. The disadvantage of transoesophageal echocardiography is that it is obviously more invasive, time-consuming and uncomfortable for the patient than

transthoracic echocardiography and it is therefore not used routinely. It is not yet part of most open access services. The main clinical problems where the technique is indicated are: endocarditis, thoracic aortic dissection (Figure 1.6), malfunctioning mitral prostheses (Figure 1.7), and transient ischaemic attack or stroke. Other possible indications are listed in Table 1.2.

Stress echocardiography

This technique is gaining ground as an alternative to nuclear myocardial perfusion

Table 1.2 Indications for transoesophageäl echocardiography

- Endocarditis
- Thoracic aortic dissection (Figure 1.6)
- Malfunction of mitral prosthesis (Figure 1.7)
- Transient ischaemic attack/stroke/ peripheral embolism
- Poor transthoracic window (but this is rare)
- Intraoperative assessment of mitral valve repair or myomectomy
- Intraoperative monitoring of left ventricular function
- Congenital disease
- Critically ill patient on intensive therapy unit
- Assessment for balloon mitral valvotomy, mitral repair or percutaneous closure of atrial septal defect

electrocardiographic exercise testing has a sensitivity and specificity of only around 60% (Mishra and Chambers, 1996). The indications for stress echocardiography are given in Table 1.3.

Further reading
Physics
Halliwell, M. Physics and principles. In Wilde, P. (ed) *Cardiac Ultrasound*. Edinburgh: Churchill Livingstone, 1993; 9–26

General books
Monaghan, M.J. *Practical Echocardiography and Doppler*. Colchester: John Wiley and Sons, 1990

Chambers, J.B. *Clinical Echocardiography*. London: BMJ Publications, 1995

Weyman, A.E. *Principles and Practice of Echocardiography*, 2nd edition. Philadelphia: Lea and Febiger, 1994

imaging (e.g. thallium, Myoview® or Cardolite® scanning). The most frequently used stressors are exercise itself or dobutamine by intravenous infusion. This mimics the physiological effects of exercise. Other pharmacological agents such as arbutamine or adenosine are also used in some centres. The technique allows the diagnosis of ischaemic heart disease, but also localises the site and quantifies the extent of ischaemia. The sensitivity in the region of 80% and specificity around 90% are comparable to those of nuclear imaging. Conventional

Table 1.3 Indications for stress echocardiography

- Clinical uncertainty and normal or equivocal conventional exercise test
- Patient unable to exercise
- Resting ECG precluding analysis (e.g. left bundle branch block, left ventricular hypertrophy with strain, digoxin)
- After acute myocardial infarction
- Need to localise site of ischaemia

Doppler ultrasound

Hatle, L. and Angelsen, B. *Doppler Ultrasound in Cardiology*, 3rd edition. Philadelphia: Lea and Febiger, 1985

Labovitz, A.J. and Williams, G.A. *Doppler Echocardiography. The Quantitative Approach*, 3rd edition. Philadelphia: Lea and Febiger, 1992

Transoesophageal echocardiography

Sutherland, G., Roelendt, J.R.T.C., Fraser, A.G. and Anderson, R.H. *Transoesophageal Echocardiography in Clinical Practice.* London: Gower Medical Publishing, 1991

Stress echo

Mishra M. and Chambers, J. Stress Echocardiography. *Br. J. Clin. Pract.* 1996 (in press)

Picano, E. *Stress Echocardiography*. Berlin: Springer Verlag, 1992

Marwick, T.H. *Stress Echocardiography.* Dordrecht: Kluwer, 1994

Chapter 2

The normal heart

Normal ranges and normal variants

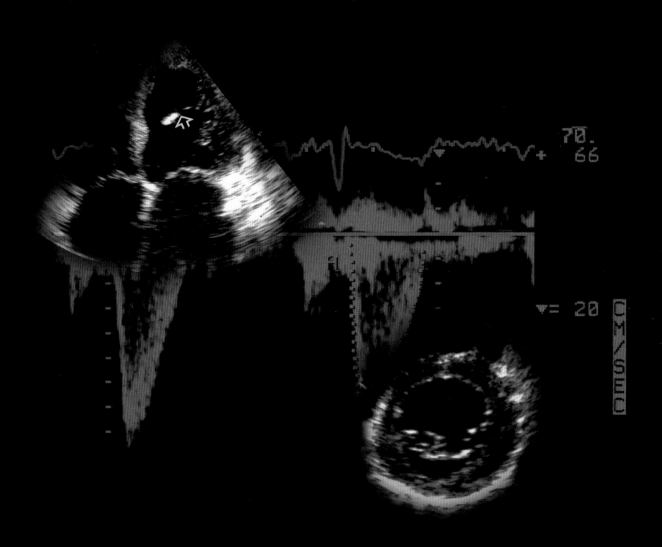

The ribs and lungs mask the heart from ultrasound except at small 'windows' (Figure 2.1) which may be enlarged by asking the subject to lie semirecumbent on his or her left side. The parasternal and apical windows are used routinely. The substernal approach is used in patients with lung disease and for imaging the

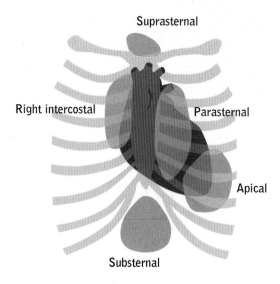

Fig 2.1 The position of the heart and the main echocardiographic 'windows'

inferior vena cava, interatrial septum and abdominal aorta; the suprasternal approach is employed mainly for imaging the aorta. The right intercostal approach is used for recording flow across the aortic valve and occasionally for specialised views, particularly of the ascending aorta.

Most examinations start with the parasternal long-axis view (Figure 2.2) in which the heart is 'sliced' lengthways from its base and towards the apex. The transducer is then rotated 90° clockwise and, by tilting on an axis between the left hip and the tip of the right shoulder, transverse (or short-axis) sections through the heart can be obtained at any level from the aorta to the apex. Three standard sections are recorded, through the aortic valve (Figure 2.3), at the level of the mitral valve (Figure 2.4), and through the papillary muscles of the left ventricle (Figure 2.5). The apical approach also allows numerous sections including a four-chamber (Figure 2.6), but also two-chamber and long-axis views. Chamber areas or derived volume are most frequently measured using the apical approach.

M-mode recordings are made at the level of the aortic cusps and through the left ventricle just below the tips of the mitral valve. Left ventricular cavity size is measured in systole and diastole (Figure 2.7). The fractional shortening is the difference between left ventricular diastolic (LVDD) and systolic dimensions (LVSD) expressed as a percentage of the diastolic dimension: $100 \times (LVDD - LVSD) / LVDD$. This is a measure of the systolic function of the base of the left ventricle but it can be used as a surrogate for the whole left ventricle provided that this has uniform shape and motion (e.g. there is no myocardial infarction or left bundle branch block).

Fig 2.2 Normal parasternal long-axis view in systole and diastole.

1 papillary muscle
2 chordae tendinae
3 anterior mitral leaflet
4 posterior mitral leaflet
5 mitral-aortic fibrosa
6 posterior mitral annulus
7 non-coronary aortic cusp
8 right coronary cusp
9 sinus of Valsalva

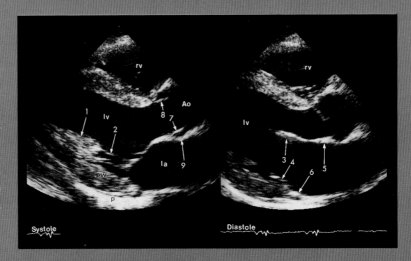

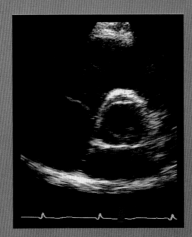

Fig 2.3 Short-axis view at aortic valve level

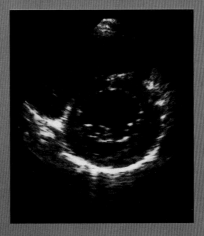

Fig 2.4 Short-axis view at mitral valve level

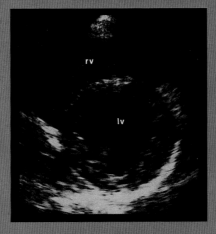

Fig 2.5 Short-axis view at papillary muscle level

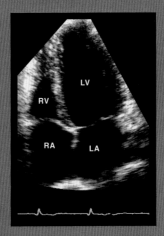

Fig 2.6 Apical four-chamber view

Fig 2.7 Measurement of cavity size on M-mode imaging. Diastolic dimensions and the aorta are measured on the Q wave. The largest left atrial and the smallest systolic left ventricular cavity dimensions are taken.

S septal width
pw posterior wall width
sd systolic LV diameter
dd diastolic LV diameter
Ao aortic diameter
LA left aortal diameter

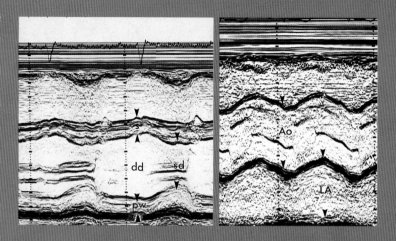

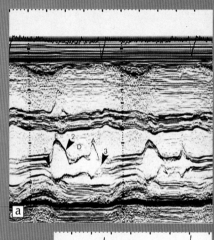

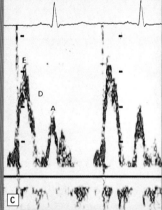

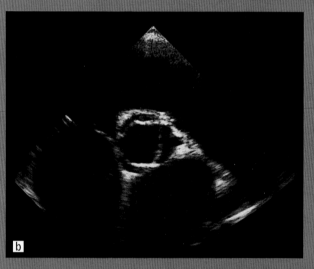

Fig 2.8 (**a**) M-mode recording at mitral valve level, (**b**) position for recording transmitral Doppler, (**c**) Transmitral Doppler.

The phases of diastole can be seen in (**a**). Initially the mitral valve leaflets open (**1**) at the start of early fast filling (**E**). The leaflets then drift towards the closed position (**2**) during diastasis (**D**) before opening again during atrial systole (**A**). After this the leaflets drift closed (**3**)

Colour flow is now turned on as a screen for abnormal flow patterns usually as a result of valve regurgitation, but occasionally from intracardiac shunts. The pulsed Doppler sample is then placed in the left ventricular cavity at the level of the tips of the mitral leaflets in their fully-open diastolic position using the four-chamber view (Figure 2.8). This gives a plot of flow velocities against time. The phases of diastole can be recorded (Figure 2.8): isovolumic relaxation before the mitral valve opens, then early active filling (E). As flow falls after this, the mitral leaflets drift towards the closed position during diastasis (D) and immediately after this the atrium contracts (A).

The sample volume is then turned to record flow through the aortic valve (Figure 2.9). The waveform is effectively a graph of velocity against time and, since distance = speed x time, the area under the curve of the waveform represents the distance travelled in one cycle by blood leaving the left ventricle. This is called the systolic velocity integral or 'stroke distance' and, when multiplied by the cross-sectional area of the left ventricular outflow tract, it gives the stroke volume. The cardiac output is then the product of stroke volume and heart rate. A complete study is recorded on videotape to allow subsequent review, re-analysis or comparison with other studies.

Normal ranges

Normal dimensions are estimated from small populations of 'average' people and may not apply in unusually small or tall subjects or in the elderly or athletic. This is potentially a major problem if echocardiography is used as a screening tool.

Traditionally, cavity dimensions are measured using M-mode which has better

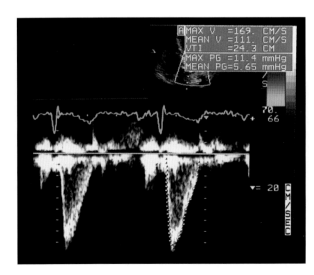

Fig 2.9 Signal recorded in the subaortic area. The pulsed Doppler sample has been placed in the left ventricular outflow tract using the apical approach. The signal has been traced around to measure systolic velocity integral (the same as stroke distance) which is 24.3 cm. Other measures automatically calculated are peak and mean velocity and derived peak and mean pressure difference

resolution than two-dimensional echocardiography. However, despite this theoretical advantage, M-mode imaging may be inaccurate unless the cursor is placed perpendicular to the structure being measured and this may not always be possible. This is frequently a problem when measuring the aortic root and left atrium when it is common to slice either structure obliquely. Similarly, right ventricular dimensions are inaccurate if measured solely in a parasternal long-axis view. Good centres will always record the scans used for calculation as well as the measurements themselves so that their accuracy can be checked retrospectively. If the cursor cannot be positioned accurately, measuremements should instead be made from the two-dimensional images. There is a good case for doing this routinely for the aortic root and left atrium. Gender-specific normal ranges for M-mode measurements are given in Table 2.1. These have been drawn up from the largest available published series and differ from the arbitrary ranges frequently adopted. In particular, the left ventricular dimensions in men are larger than commonly appreciated. Thus, mild dilated myopathy should not be diagnosed on the basis of an apparently large cavity size alone. Another frequent error is to overestimate the posterior wall width by incorporating chordal echoes in the measurement. Left ventricular hypertrophy should rarely be diagnosed from this measurement alone. Normal ranges for two-dimensional dimensions are given in Figure 2.10. If an accurate assessment of aortic size is required, this should be performed using two-dimensional rather than M-mode echocardiography using the levels shown in Figure 2.11. Normal ranges for aortic size are given in Table 2.2.

Intracardiac dimensions are related to body size and in 'outsize' individuals, it may be difficult to decide if a cavity dimension is normal. It is traditional to index these to body surface area (BSA)

Table 2.1 Normal intracardiac dimensions (cm) in men and women aged 18–72 years, 150–203 cm (59–80 ins) in height

	Men		Women	
Left atrium	3.0 – 4.5	$n = 288$	2.7 – 4.0	$n = 524$
LV diastolic diameter	4.3 – 5.9	$n = 394$	4.0 – 5.2	$n = 643$
LV systolic diameter	2.6 – 4.0	$n = 288$	2.3 – 3.5	$n = 524$
IV septum (diastole)	0.6 – 1.3	$n = 106$	0.5 – 1.2	$n = 109$
Posterior wall (diastole)	0.6 – 1.2	$n = 106$	0.5 – 1.1	$n = 119$

References: Lauer, M.S. *et al. JACC* 1995; **26**; 1039–46 Devereux, R.B. *et al. JACC* 1984; **4**: 1222–30
LV=left ventricular   IV=interventricular and intraventricular

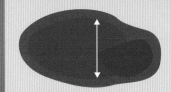

D 3.4–5.3 cm
S 2.3–4.4 cm

D 3.5–6.1 cm
S 2.3–4.1 cm

D 3.9–5.9 cm
S 2.7–4.9 cm

Fig 2.10 Normal ranges
for two-dimensional dimensions.
D diastole, **S** systole

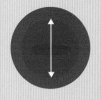

D 3.7–6.0 cm
S 2.6–4.4 cm

D 5.9–9.0 cm
S 4.5–7.9 cm

Reference: Pearlman, J.D. *et al.* Limits of
normal left ventricular dimensions in growth
and development: analysis of dimensions and
variance in the two-dimensional
echocardiograms of 268 normal healthy
subjects. *JACC* 1988; **12**: 1432–41

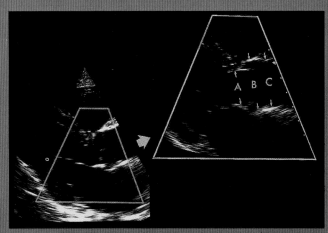

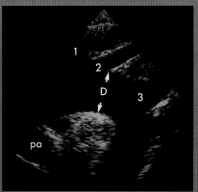

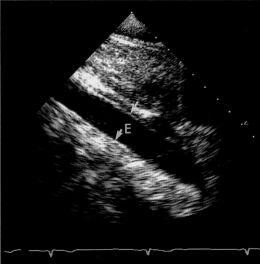

Fig 2.11 The aorta showing
levels for measurement

A annulus
B sinus of Valsalva
C sinotubular junction
D arch
E abdominal aorta
pa pulmonary artery
1 the innominate artery
2 the left carotid
3 the left subclavian artery

although there is good evidence that some dimensions such as the aortic root diameter are better related to height (Nidorf, 1992). M-mode dimensions are given in relation to height in Table 2.3 and two-dimensional dimensions in relation to BSA in Table 2.4. For these data, the DuBois method of calculating BSA was used, but a convenient alternative method (Mosteller, 1987) for clinical use is:

$$BSA = \sqrt{(\text{height in cm} \times \text{weight in kg}/3600)}$$

The elderly are another difficult group since it is not clear whether variations are strictly normal or represent the effect of

Table 2.2 Normal ranges (95% confidence intervals) for aortic diameter (cm) using two-dimensional echocardiography

Level (Figure 2.11)	Sample size	Absolute	Indexed to body surface area
A Annulus	n = 195	1.7 – 2.5	1.1 – 1.5 [1,2,3]
B Sinus of Valsalva	n = 39	2.2 – 3.6	1.4 – 2.0 [4]
C Sinotubular junction	n = 26	1.8 – 2.6	1.0 – 1.6 [5]
D Arch	n = 47	1.4 – 2.9	0.8 – 1.9 [1]
E Abdominal aorta	n = 50	1.0 – 2.2	0.6 – 1.3 [1]

References: 1. Guy's database   2. Oh, J.K. et al. JACC 1988; **11**: 1227–34   3. Davidson, W.R. et al. Am. J. Cardiol. 1991; **67**: 547–9
4. Schnittger, I. et al. JACC 1983; **5**: 934–8   5. Mintz, G.S. et al. Am. J. Cardiol. 1979; **44**: 232–8

Table 2.3 Upper limit of intracardiac dimensions (cm) by height (m)

Height	1.41–1.45	1.46–1.50	1.51–1.55	1.56–1.60	1.61–1.65	1.66–1.70	1.71–1.75	1.76–1.80	1.81–1.85	1.86–1.90	>1.90
M-mode											
Male											
LVDD			5.3	5.4	5.5	5.5	5.6	5.7	5.8	5.9	>6.0
LVSD			3.6	3.7	3.7	3.8	3.8	3.9	3.9	4.0	>4.0
Female											
LVDD	4.9	4.9	5.0	5.1	5.1	5.2	5.3	5.3			
LVSD	3.1	3.2	3.3	3.3	3.4	3.4	3.5	3.5			
Two-dimensional											
Ann	2.0	2.0	2.1	2.1	2.2	2.2	2.3	2.3	2.4	2.4	>2.4
LA	3.2	3.3	3.4	3.4	3.5	3.6	3.6	3.7	3.8	3.9	>3.9

References: Lauer, M.S. et al. JACC 1995; **26**; 1039–46   Nidorf, S.M. et al. JACC 1992; **19**: 983–8
Ann = aortic annulus   LA = left atrium   LVDD = left ventricular diastolic dimension   LVSD = left ventricular systolic dimension

Table 2.4 Intracardiac dimensions (cm) on two-dimensional echocardiography by body surface area

| | | Body surface area (m²) | | |
		1.4–1.6	1.6–1.8	1.8–2.0
Parasternal long-axis	Diastole	3.4–4.9	3.6–5.1	3.9–5.3
	Systole	2.3–3.9	2.4–4.1	2.5–4.4
Parasternal short-axis mitral level	Diastole	3.7–5.4	3.9–5.7	4.1–6.0
	Systole	2.6–4.0	2.8–4.3	2.9–4.4
Parasternal short-axis papillary	Diastole	3.5–5.5	3.8–5.8	4.1–6.1
	Systole	2.3–3.9	2.4–4.0	2.6–4.1
Four-chamber mediolateral	Diastole	3.9–5.4	4.0–5.6	4.1–5.9
	Systole	2.7–4.5	2.9–4.7	3.1–4.9
Four-chamber long-axis	Diastole	5.9–8.3	6.3–8.7	6.6–9.0
	Systole	4.5–6.9	4.6–7.4	4.6–7.9

Reference: Pearlman, J.D. *et al. JACC* 1988; **12**: 1432–41

Table 2.5 Effect of age on diameter of ascending aorta (cm)

| | | Height (m) | | |
Site	Age (years)	1.4–1.6	1.6–1.8	1.8–2.0
Sinus of Valsalva	<40	2.1–3.2	2.3–3.4	2.5–3.6
	>40	2.3–3.8	2.3–4.0	2.5–4.3
Sinotubular junction	<40	1.9–2.8	2.0–3.0	2.1–3.1
	>40	2.1–3.3	2.1–3.5	2.1–3.6

Reference: Roman, M.J. *et al. Am. J. Cardiol.* 1989; **64**: 507–12

occult or long-standing mild disease such as hypertension or coronary disease. The elderly tend to have thicker septal and posterior wall widths, but a thickness greater than 1.3 cm is usually abnormal (Klein, 1994). Chamber dimensions are variously reported as larger (Pearson, 1991)

or smaller (Klein, 1994) than average, possibly reflecting the presence of different disease states. The aorta is affected by age differently at each level. The annulus is not affected whilst the sinus of Valsalva and sinotubular junction increase in size significantly with age (Table 2.5).

Table 2.6 Cardiac dimensions (cm) in athletic individuals (95% confidence limits)

	Male ($n = 738$)	Female ($n = 209$)
LA	3.1–4.3	2.8–4.0
LVDD	4.6–6.2	4.1–5.6
IVS	0.8–1.3	0.7–1.0
PW	0.8–1.1	0.6–1.1

Reference: Pelliccia, A. *et al. N. Engl. J. Med.* 1991; **324**; 295–301
LA = left atrium   LVDD = left ventricular diastolic dimension   IVS = interventricular septum
PW = posterior wall

Table 2.7 Great vessel peak velocities of blood flow in 110 normal subjects

Site	95% limits (m/s)
Ascending aorta	0.66–1.42
Descending aorta	0.67–1.35
Abdominal aorta	0.47–1.67
Pulmonary artery	0.48–1.16

Reference: Wilson, N. *Br. Heart J.* 1985; **53**: 451–8

Active athletic individuals may also cause diagnostic confusion. Except in weight lifters, the heart in a trained athlete is slightly dilated and mildly hypertrophied. The septal width is rarely >1.3 cm and probably never >1.6 cm, but the diastolic cavity dimension may be up to 6.2 cm (Pelliccia, 1991) (Table 2.6). Because it habitually performs at high preload, the left ventricle may be relatively hypocontractile at rest. It is easy to overdiagnose a mild dilated cardiomyopathy in these people. What constitutes athleticism is inevitably open to question, but borderline hypocontractility with a fractional shortening around 25% in a healthy active person is likely to be normal.

Normal ranges for Doppler velocities are given in Table 2.7. Relatively high velocities are found in patients with high cardiac output as a result of fever, anaemia, pregnancy or anxiety. Ascending aortic velocities of 2.0 m/s are frequently found. Transmitral filling velocities are described in Chapter 3.

Normal variants and technical problems

Most normal variants are obvious but, in the search for pathology in otherwise normal people, these may cause confusion. A large eustachian valve (Figure 2.12) or left ventricular tendon (Figure 2.13) are normal variants which are occasionally misinterpreted as masses. Reverberation artefact (Figure 2.14) may also be overinterpreted as a mass. Technical errors can occur from fore-shortening the apex or measuring septal width through a right ventricular papillary muscle to mimic hypertrophy. Another problem is the faithful reporting of small jets of regurgitation, which, to the uninitiated, may suggest pathology In fact, ultrasound

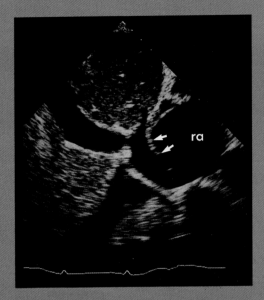

Fig 2.12 Normal variant :
large eustachian valve. This valve
guards the opening of the inferior
vena cava into the right atrium

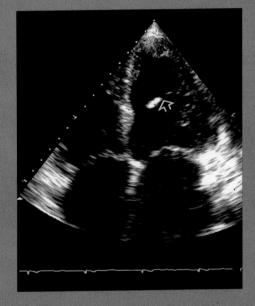

Fig 2.13 Normal variant:
left ventricular tendon

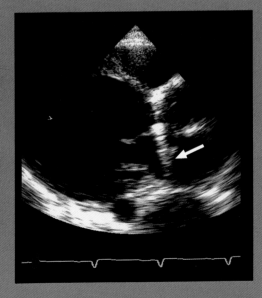

Fig 2.14 Artefact:
reverberation artefact
from a mechanical
prosthetic valve in the
aortic position causes the
appearance of echoes
within the left atrium
(arrow) which may be
mistaken for a mass

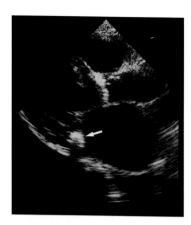

Fig 2.15 Posterior mitral annular calcification (arrow)

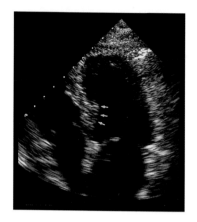

Fig 2.16 Normal variant: localised subaortic bulge (arrows)

machines are now so sensitive that trivial tricuspid and pulmonary regurgitation are found in virtually all normal subjects and trivial mitral regurgitation may be found in around one-third. However, minor aortic regurgitation is unusual and likely to be abnormal.

Age-related changes should not be overinterpreted. Minor aortic valve thickening is very frequent and not in itself a sign of significant pathology. Mitral annular calcification (Figure 2.15) is occasionally misinterpreted as a vegetation, thrombus or myxoma. Localised subaortic bulging of the septum (Figure 2.16) is normal in the elderly and should not be diagnosed as hypertrophic cardiomyopathy.

References

Klein, A.L., Burstow, D.J., Tajik, A.J., Zachariah, P.K., Bailey, K.R. and Seward, J.B. Effects of age on left ventricular dimensions and filling dynamics in 117 normal persons. *Mayo Clin. Proc.* 1994; **69**: 212–24

Mosteller, R.D. Simplified calculation of body surface area. *N. Engl. J. Med.* 1987; **317**: 1098

Nidorf, S.M., Picard, M.H., Triulzi, M.O., Thomas, J.D., Newell, J., King, M.E. and Weyman, A.E. New perspectives in the assessment of cardiac chamber dimensions during development and adulthood. *JACC* 1992; **19**: 983–8

Pelliccia, A., Maron, B.J., Spataro, A., Proschan, M.A. and Spirito, P. The upper limit of physiologic cardiac hypertrophy in highly trained elite athletes. *N. Engl. J. Med.* 1991; **324**; 295–301

Pearson, A.C., Gudipati, C., Nagelhout, D., Sear, J., Cohen, J.D., Labovitz, A.J. and technical assistance of Mrosek, D. and Vrain, J. St. Echocardiographic evaluation of cardiac structure and function in elderly subjects with isolated hypertension. *JACC* 1991; **17**: 422–30

Schiller, N.B., Shah, P.M., Crawford, M., DeMaria, A., Devereux, R., Feigenbaum, H., Gutgesell, H., Reichek, N., Sahn, D., Schnittger, I., Silverman, N.H. and Tajik, A.J. Recommendations for quantitation of the left ventricle by two-dimensional echocardiography. *Am. Soc. Echo.* 1989; **2**: 358–67

Chapter 3

Suspected heart failure

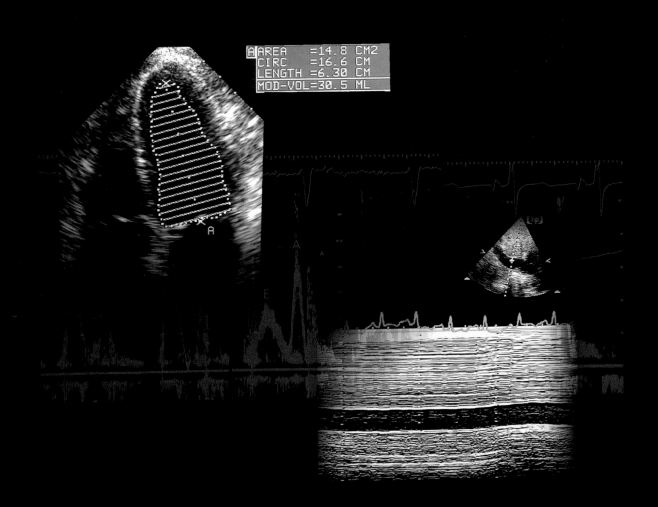

Heart failure is not in itself a complete diagnosis. The aetiology and underlying pathophysiological mechanisms need to be determined, as these may affect treatment. For example, as many as 3% of people aged over 75 years may have severe aortic stenosis (Lindroos, 1993). If this causes heart failure, the murmur may become inaudible. Approximately one-third of patients with clinical heart failure have predominantly diastolic rather than systolic left ventricular dysfunction (Soufer, 1985). In both these instances, angiotensin converting enzyme (ACE) inhibitors may be either unhelpful or dangerous.

myocardial infarct, dominant systolic dysfunction can be assumed and conventional treatment with diuretics and ACE inhibitors instituted. Echocardiography is necessary if the diagnosis of heart failure is not proved and either the aetiology or pathophysiology is uncertain. Although these are two separate entities, they may be closely linked. For example the presence of a hypertrophied, but normally-contracting left ventricle strongly suggests an aetiology (hypertrophic cardiomyopathy or hypertension) and the pathophysiology (diastolic dysfunction).

The echocardiogram is also used to exclude conditions that mimic heart failure or require specific therapy other than diuretics and ACE inhibitors. For example, valve disease or left ventricular aneurysm may require surgery.

Table 3.1 Indications for echocardiography in suspected heart failure
Widely accepted
• Unexplained breathlessness
• Clinical signs of heart failure (third sound, high jugular venous pressure, basal crackles), but aetiology not established
In discussion
• Currently treated with antifailure drugs
• Asymptomatic but at risk of left ventricular dysfunction e.g. post myocardial infarction

Heart failure is common, with an annual incidence of around 0.8 cases per 1000 people aged over 65 years (Cowie, 1996). This would represent a vast load if every case required echocardiography. Thankfully, ischaemic disease is the most likely aetiology. Thus, if a patient has clinical heart failure and a documented

Establishing the diagnosis and pathophysiology

Initially, the echocardiographer excludes valve disease as a cause of breathlessness or secondary heart failure. Other conditions that mimic heart failure, such as pericardial effusion (Figure 3.1) or left atrial myxoma, must also be looked for. The diagnosis is then made by establishing evidence of significant systolic or diastolic dysfunction.

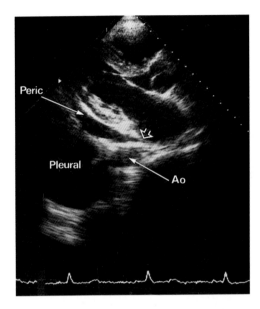

Fig 3.1 Pericardial and pleural effusions. These can be differentiated from the relative position of the descending thoracic aorta. The pericardial effusion finishes anterior (arrow) and the pleural effusion posterior to the descending aorta (Ao)

Systolic function

Both regional and global systolic function are examined. Every region corresponding to the arterial supply of the heart (Figure 3.2) is described according to the degree of systolic thickening and by the motion of the endocardium:

- normal
- hypokinetic (the endocardium moves inwards less than 50% of normal) (Figure 3.3)
- akinetic (no motion)
- dyskinetic (motion out of phase with the expected direction) (Figure 3.4).

Global measures of function include ejection fraction, stroke volume, and

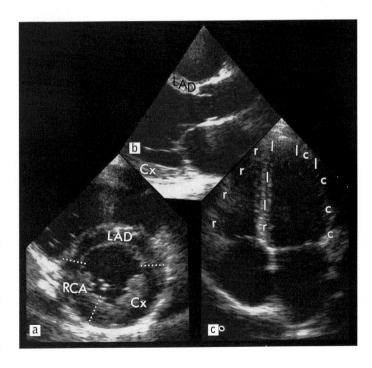

Fig 3.2 The arterial supply of the heart shown in parasternal short axis (**a**), long axis (**b**), and four-chamber (**c**) views. Note: in (**c**) r = right coronary artery; l = left anterior descending; c = circumflex

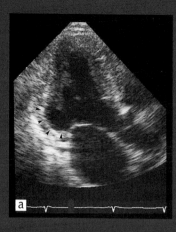

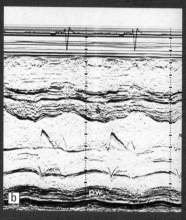

Fig 3.3 Hypokinesis. There is an inferior infarct shown as a bulging region (arrowed in **a**). The M-mode recording at this level (**b**) shows hyperkinesis of the septum (**s**) while the inferior wall (**pw**) is hypokinetic

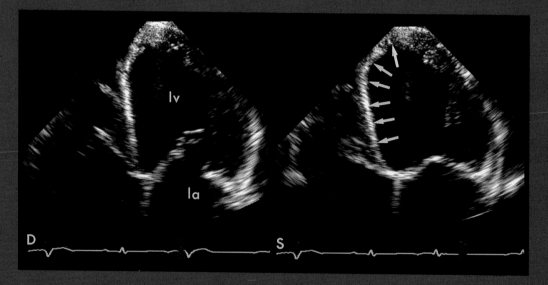

Fig 3.4 Anterior myocardial infarct. The apex and adjacent septum are thin and move paradoxically, i.e. outwards in systole (right, arrows) when the rest of the left ventricle is moving inwards. Note: **D** = diastole; **S** = systole

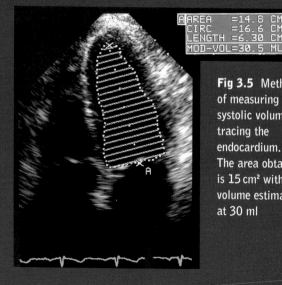

Fig 3.5 Method of measuring end-systolic volume by tracing the endocardium. The area obtained is 15 cm² with a volume estimated at 30 ml

end-systolic volume. Ejection fraction is usually estimated by eye, but can also be calculated using online computer software. This involves tracing round systolic and diastolic frames usually in the apical four-chamber and two-chamber views. Systolic and diastolic volumes are calculated using geometric assumptions (Figure 3.5). Stroke volume is then the difference between diastolic and systolic volume and ejection fraction is stroke volume expressed as a percentage of the diastolic volume. Normal ranges are given in Table 3.2. However these calculations are laborious and potentially inaccurate. End-systolic chamber area or derived-volume alone are relatively more accurate because, for technical reasons, the endocardium is well-imaged in systole. In the diseased heart, there is often a change in shape of the left ventricular cavity even if there is no regional abnormality of

Table 3.2 Normal ranges (95% confidence limits) for measures of systolic and diastolic function

Echocardiography		
Fractional shortening (%)	28–44	
End-diastolic volume (ml)*	58–166 (male)	49–129 (female)
End-systolic volume (ml)*	3–67 (male)	9–57 (female)
Four-chamber area diastole (cm²)	18.6–48.6	
Four-chamber area systole (cm²)	8.6–30.4	
Ejection fraction (%)	50–70	
Doppler		
Systolic velocity integral (cm)	15–35	10–25 (elderly)
Mitral valve E (cm/s)	44–100	34–90 (elderly)
Mitral valve A (cm/s)	20–60	31–87 (elderly)
E:A ratio	0.7–3.1	0.5–1.7 (elderly)
Tricuspid valve E (cm/s)	20–50	
Tricuspid valve A (cm/s)	12–36	
E:A ratio	0.8–2.9	
Time intervals		
Mitral E deceleration time (ms)	139–219	138–282 (elderly)
Mitral A deceleration time (ms)	>70	
Isovolumic relaxation time (ms)	54–98	56–124 (elderly)

References: Van Dam, I. *et al. Echocardiography* 1988; **5**: 259–67 Zarich, S.W. *et al. JACC* 1988; **12**: 114–30 Wilson, N. *et al. Br. Heart J.* 1985; **53**; 451–8 Wahr, D.W. *et al. JACC* 1983; **1**: 863–8 Schiller, N.B. and Foster, E. *Heart* 1996; **75** (Suppl 2): 17–26 Sagie, A. *et al. J. Am. Soc. Echo* 1993; **6**: 570–6 Van Dam, I. *Eur. Heart J.* 1988; **9**: 165–71 Klein, A.L. *et al. Mayo Clin. Proc.* 1994; **69**: 212–24 Rawles, J. *Echocardiography: an International Review.* 1993; 23–36 Pearlman, J.D. *JACC* 1988; **12**: 1432–41

* Single plane four-chamber view

movement. Therefore, these end-systolic quantities often reflect the true size of the heart better than do M-mode dimensions. Stroke volume can also be calculated from the product of the cross-sectional area of the aorta and the area of the pulsed Doppler signal recorded in the left ventricular outflow tract (Figure 3.6). This is accurate and compares favourably with thermodilution methods.

Diastolic dysfunction

Diastolic dysfunction is suggested by the presence of left ventricular hypertrophy in a patient with breathlessness or by abrupt cessation of filling shown as a jerky diastolic motion on two-dimensional imaging. More specific evidence is found from abnormalities of transmitral flow recorded using pulsed Doppler (Figure 3.7). In the normal person, the early velocity (E wave) is higher than the velocity during atrial systole (A wave) and the E descent is quick. There are two main pathological patterns (Figure 3.7). The first is called the 'slow relaxation pattern' and consists of a low E wave, prolonged E wave deceleration time (and isovolumic relaxation time) with a tall A wave. This pattern is seen in hypertrophied left ventricles. The second pattern is the 'restrictive pattern' which occurs in left ventricular dysfunction from any cause associated with high filling pressures (pulmonary wedge pressure > 20 mmHg) or with a fast rate of rise of left ventricular diastolic pressure (as in restrictive myopathy

or pericardial constriction). This has a tall E wave, short E deceleration time (and short isovolumic relaxation time) with a small or absent A wave. Other signs of abnormal diastolic function are a dilated inferior vena cava or abnormal patterns of pulmonary, superior vena cava or hepatic vein flow. For example an abnormally increased peak velocity or duration of atrial flow reversal on pulmonary venous flow recordings suggests elevated end-diastolic left ventricular pressure.

Surgically correctable diseases, mainly pericardial constriction must first be excluded by advanced echocardiographic techniques, sometimes supplemented by computed tomography or even cardiac catheterisation. Treatment is then with diuretics and, with specialist advice, drugs which reduce the heart rate or speed of relaxation. These include beta blockers and verapamil. ACE inhibitors are usually unhelpful or harmful in pure diastolic heart failure.

Right-sided disease

Right-sided failure is shown by a dilated, hypokinetic right ventricle. This may be difficult to detect, but, if the right ventricle is the same size or larger than the left ventricle in all views, it must be abnormal. Dilatation of the inferior vena cava (Figure 3.8) is a sign of high right-sided pressures as a non-specific sign of left or right ventricular failure or pericardial disease.

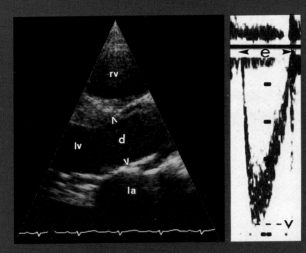

Fig 3.6 Method of estimating stroke volume. This is calculated from the product of the cross-sectional area of the left ventricular outflow tract and the area of the subaortic signal recorded using pulsed Doppler (stroke distance or systolic velocity integral). Note: **d** = diameter; **e** = ejection time; **v** = peak velocity

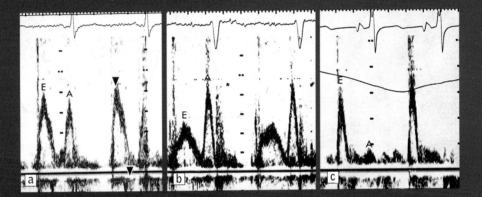

Fig 3.7 Transmitral pulsed Doppler recordings. These were all recorded with the sample volume positioned as shown in Fig 2.8. The patterns are normal (**a**), slow filling (**b**), and restrictive (**c**). The method of measuring the deceleration time of the E wave is shown in **a** (between the two arrows)

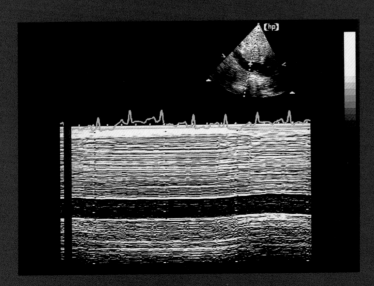

Fig 3.8 Dilated inferior vena cava. The diameter should be less than 2 cm and there should be constriction by at least 50% during inspiration. In this image, the diameter remains constant. This is a non-specific sign of a raised right atrial pressure, in this case caused by pericardial constriction

Table 3.3 Significant left ventricular dysfunction suggesting that heart failure is the likely cause of symptoms

a Systolic abnormalities

- ejection fraction <40%
- end-systolic volume >70 ml or 45 ml/m²
- fractional shortening <20%
- stroke distance <10 cm
- extensive regional wall motion abnormality

b Diastolic abnormalities

- mitral E wave deceleration time <100 ms
- mitral A wave deceleration time <60 ms

Can we define criteria for diagnosing heart failure?

There are no simple universal criteria and these will depend on the level of suspicion based on the clinical findings. The presence of clinical signs of heart failure and the absence of other causes of breathlessness suggests a high clinical suspicion of heart failure. The presence of breathlessness alone denotes a lower level of suspicion and demands a higher grade of abnormality on the echocardiogram before a working diagnosis of heart failure should be made. Tables 3.3 and 3.4 give guidelines for determining the likelihood of clinical heart failure. These are to some degree arbitrary, but are based on normal ranges.

If clinical doubt remains, the patient must be seen by a cardiologist. **In the presence of a normal echocardiogram, the heart may still be a cause for breathlessness as a result of systolic failure on exertion, occult diastolic dysfunction, or angina.** Diastolic dysfunction is difficult to diagnose except by experienced echocardiographers. An apparently normal left ventricle on superficial examination may still be the cause of breathlessness.

Table 3.4 Heart failure is a possible cause of breathlessness

a Systolic abnormalities

- ejection fraction 40–50%
- fractional shortening 20–25%
- stroke distance 10–15 cm

b Diastolic abnormalities

- mitral E wave deceleration time >280 ms or <140 ms
- mitral A wave deceleration time <70 ms
- increased left ventricular mass 134 g/m² in men and 110 g/m² in women
- E:A ratio <1.0
- increased velocity and duration of pulmonary vein flow reversal during atrial systole

Screening for occult left ventricular dysfunction

There is evidence that patients with left ventricular dilatation or reduced contractility have a higher than average risk of death (Lauer, 1992). There is also evidence that patients after acute myocardial infarction with impaired left ventricles defined by nuclear scanning (Pfeffer, 1992) or by wall motion analysis (Kobler, 1995) may benefit from ACE inhibitors. However, results using ejection fraction by nuclear ventriculography cannot reliably be extrapolated to echocardiography (Ray, 1995) and there are no studies justifying the treatment of patients with occult left ventricular impairment late rather than early after infarction or from causes other than ischaemic disease. It remains premature to screen the population at risk to detect occult dysfunction.

Should all patients on antifailure medication be screened?

Preliminary reports suggest that over one-half of all patients taking diuretics or ACE inhibitors have no evidence of a left ventricular systolic abnormality at rest (Francis, 1995). Allowing for cases with hypertension or ankle oedema, treatment with diuretics was judged to be inappropriate in 44% of cases in one study (Francis, 1995). However, this underplays the importance of diastolic dysfunction. Furthermore, the echocardiogram may not always reflect the pretreatment state of the patient. Minor abnormalities of systolic or diastolic function may not be obvious at rest or may be obscured by drug treatment. The drug may even have corrected an underlying abnormality as, for example, when an ACE inhibitor induces regression of left ventricular hypertrophy. Ideally, the whole clinical history should be reviewed checking for previously documented objective signs, evidence of improvement on therapy, other possible causes of breathlessness or other explanations for clinical signs (e.g. varicose veins for ankle swelling). The echocardiogram should be part of this general clinical review, but should not replace it.

Does a normal electrocardiogram exclude the need for echocardiography?

Recent reports have suggested that it is rare to have an abnormal echocardiogram in the presence of a normal electrocardiogram (Francis, 1996). Despite their suggestion that echocardiography is not necessary if the electrocardiogram is normal, some 10–15% of patients with normal electrocardiograms have important systolic dysfunction on echocardiography. Furthermore, these studies fail to take account of the frequency of diastolic dysfunction. A common cause of this is left ventricular hypertrophy as a result of hypertension and it is already well-documented that echocardiography is 5–10 times more sensitive than electrocardiography for the detection of left ventricular hypertrophy (see Chapter 5).

I suggest that an electrocardiogram is a useful first investigation in patients with breathlessness or clinical heart failure. It may show an arrhythmia such as uncontrolled atrial fibrillation as a likely cause of the symptoms. It may also show the signs of a myocardial infarction in which case the clinician is on firm ground in treating with diuretics and ACE inhibitors. In the absence of overt heart failure, the possibility of angina must always be considered in such patients. However, it is precisely those patients with no electrocardiographic abnormalities or who have equivocal or non-specific ST/T wave changes where echocardiography is likely to be most helpful in detecting heart failure and in determining the aetiology.

Aetiology of heart failure

The most frequent aetiologies of heart failure are ischaemic disease, hypertension, valve disease, and high alcohol consumption. Ischaemic heart disease is characterised by regional wall motion abnormalities (Figure 3.4). There may be complications of infarction such as left ventricular aneurysm (Figure 3.9) or, rarely, ventricular septal rupture which is present in 1–2% of all acute infarcts. Hypertensive heart disease is suggested by increased left ventricular mass (see Chapter 5) with either a small or dilated

cavity depending on the stage of disease, individual susceptibility to pressure overload and, possibly, the presence of coronary disease. Hypertrophic cardiomyopathy is a possibility if there is significant hypertrophy (septal width >1.5 cm) (Figure 3.10) with no history of hypertension. Dilated cardiomyopathy is shown by an unthickened, dilated, globally hypocontractile ventricle (Figure 3.11). However, idiopathic dilated cardiomyopathy cannot be distinguished echocardiographically from specific causes of left ventricular disease such as high alcohol consumption.

Left ventricular dysfunction secondary to valve disease is easily detected by the presence of anatomical abnormalities of the valve on two-dimensional imaging, together with significant aortic stenosis or aortic or mitral regurgitation on continuous wave Doppler. The differentiation between severe mitral regurgitation causing left ventricular failure and primary left ventricular myopathy associated with significant functional mitral regurgitation may be difficult. If systolic function is severely impaired with a fractional shortening <29% (or end-systolic volume >90 ml/m^2) the distinction is in any case largely academic since valve surgery is unlikely to reverse left ventricular dysfunction (Ross, 1985). It is important to remember that in the presence of severe mitral regurgitation, the fractional

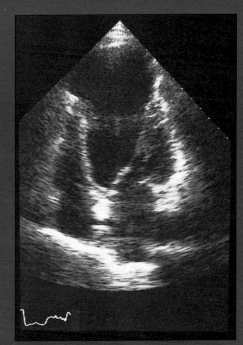

Fig 3.9 Left ventricular aneurysm. There is a large bulge with a wide neck at the apex of the left ventricle

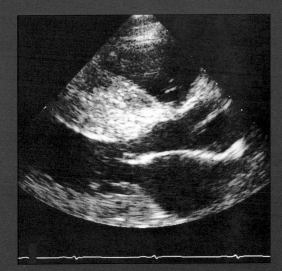

Fig 3.10 Hypertrophic cardiomyopathy. This parasternal long-axis view shows a severely hypertrophied septum

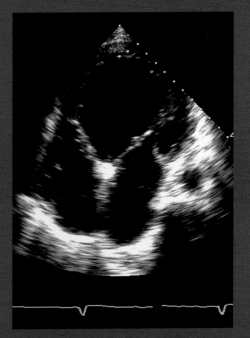

Fig 3.11 Dilated left ventricle in an apical four-chamber view

Fig 3.12 M-mode recordings through the left ventricle before and after mitral valve surgery. The fractional shortening before surgery (**a**) was 29% and afterwards (**b**) was 15%

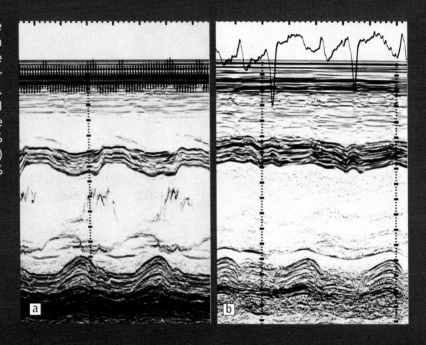

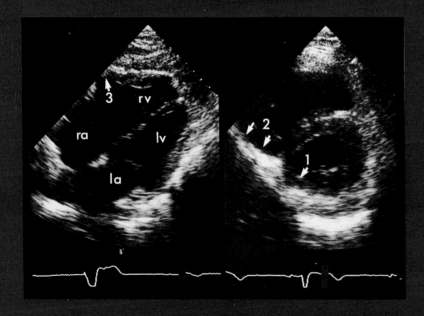

Fig 3.13 Right ventricular infarction. There is an infarct of the inferior wall of the left ventricle (**1**) with thinning and akinesis of the adjacent part of the right ventricle (**2**). The base of the free wall is also affected (**3**)

shortening may be normal despite intrinsically reduced contractility. This is because the ventricle contracts into the left atrium which offers much less resistance than the aorta. It is a little like being treated with large doses of ACE inhibitors. After mitral valve surgery, the left ventricle is then subject to normal afterload and its fractional shortening may fall (Figure 3.12).

A combination of two-dimensional imaging and Doppler findings can also detect the causes of right ventricular dysfunction, namely pulmonary hypertension, intracardiac shunts, right-sided valve disease, right ventricular infarction (Figure 3.13), and right ventricular cardiomyopathy.

References

Cowie, M.R., Penston, H., Wood, D.A., Coats, A., Thompson, S., Poole-Wilson, P.A. and Sutton, G.C. A population-based survey of the incidence of heart failure. *Heart* 1996; **73** (Suppl 1): P38 (Abstract)

Francis, C.M., Davie, A., Sutherland, G.R. and McMurray, J.J.V. A normal electrocardiogram predicts normal left ventricular systolic function in patients with suspected heart failure. *Heart* 1995; **73** (Suppl 3): 14 (Abstract)

Francis, C.M., Caruàna, L., Kearney, P., Love, M., Sutherland, G.R., Starkey, I.R. and Shaw, T.R.D. Open access echocardiography in management of heart failure in the community. *Br. Med. J.* 1995; **310**: 634–6

Køber, L., Torp-Pedersen, C., Carlsen, J.E., Bagger, H., Eliasen, P., Lynnborg, K., Videbek, J.,

Cole, D.S., Auclert, L., Pauly, N.C., Aliot, E., Persson, S. and Camm, A.J. A clinical trial of the angiotensin-converting enzyme inhibitor Trandolapril in patients with left ventricular dysfunction after myocardial infarction. *N. Engl. J. Med.* 1995; **333**: 1670–6

Lauer, M.S., Evans, J.C. and Levy, D. Prognostic implications of subclinical left ventricular dilatation and systolic dysfunction in men free of overt cardiovascular disease (the Framingham Heart Study). *Am. J. Cardiol.* 1992; **70**: 1180–4

Lindroos, M., Kupari, M., Heikkilä, J. and Tilvis, R. Prevalence of aortic valve abnormalities in the elderly: an echocardiographic study of a random population sample. *JACC* 1993; **21**: 1220–5

Little, W.C. and Downes, T.R. The clinical evaluation of left ventricular diastolic performance. *Progress in Cardiovascular Disease* 1990; **32**: 273–90

Pfeffer, M.A., Braunwald, E., Moyé, L.A., Basta, L., Brown, E.J., Cuddy, T.E., Davis, B.R., Geltman, E.M., Goldman, S., Flaker, G.C., Klein, M., Lamas, G.A., Packer, M., Rouleau, J., Rouleau, J.L., Rutherford, J., Wertheimer, J.H. and Hawkins, C.M. Effect of captopril on mortality and morbidity in patients with left ventricular dysfunction after myocardial infarction. *N. Engl. J. Med.* 1992; **327**: 669–77

Ray, S.G., Metcalfe, M.J., Oldroyd, K.G., Pye, M., Martin, W., Christie, J., Dargie, H.J. and Cobbe, S.M. Do radionuclide and echocardiographic techniques give a universal cut off value for left ventricular ejection fraction that can be used to select patients for treatment with ACE inhibitors after myocardial infarction? *Br. Heart J.* 1995; **73**: 466–9

Ross, J. Afterload mismatch in aortic and mitral valve disease; implication for surgical therapy. *JACC* 1985; **5**: 811–26

Soufer, R., Wohlgelernter, D., Vita, N.A., Amuchestegui, M., Sostman, A.D. and Berger, H.L. Intact systolic left ventricular function in clinical congestive heart failure. *Am. J. Cardiol.* 1985; **55**: 1032–6

Chapter 4

The patient
with a murmur

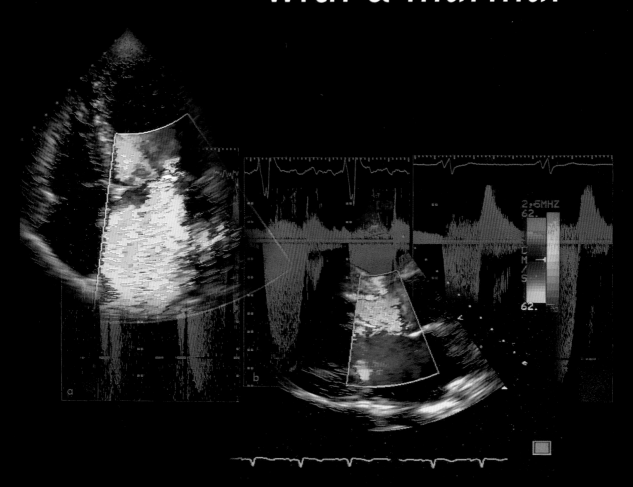

Murmurs are caused by valve disease, an intracardiac shunt, or high flow across a normal valve. Echocardiography is necessary if there is the possibility of significant disease (Table 4.1) or to check if antibiotic prophylaxis is necessary. It confirms the site of origin of the murmur by imaging an abnormal valve or detecting abnormal flow on colour mapping. It can then reveal the aetiology and quantify the severity of disease.

Table 4.1 Indications for echocardiography in patients with a murmur

- Ejection systolic murmur and one of the following:
  - chest pain, breathlessness or dizzy spells on exertion
  - evidence of strain on electrocardiogram
  - heart failure
- Ejection murmur filling most of systole or with a soft second sound
- Any diastolic murmur
- Any pansystolic murmur
- Abnormal second heart sound
- Wide pulse pressure and displaced apex beat or enlarged cardiac shadow
- Suspicion of acute aortic dissection or endocarditis

Note: Asymptomatic patients with a short, soft ejection systolic murmur and an easily heard second sound which splits normally do not require echocardiography

Aetiology

The most frequent cause of aortic stenosis in western populations is calcific degenerative disease (Figure 4.1). Minor thickening of the aortic valve is found in 20% of all people aged over 65 years and 40% aged over 75 years (Lindroos, 1993). This explains why a short, soft systolic murmur should not automatically require echocardiography. Mild aortic thickening may progress, so the term 'aortic sclerosis' should be avoided as this is often taken to imply a separate, more benign aetiology. A bicuspid aortic valve occurs in around 2% of the population (Figure 4.2), and usually results from failure of two of the cusps to separate during embryological development. The valve is subject to increased strain and thickens and calcifies more rapidly than usual leading to significant aortic stenosis typically between 40 and 60 years of age. Aortic regurgitation can be caused either by dilatation of the aortic root or by aortic valve disease, or both. In western populations, aortic root dilatation (Figure 4.3) is the more frequent cause of significant regurgitation. It usually develops as a result of arteriosclerosis secondary to ageing. Of the valve-related causes of regurgitation, rheumatic disease tends to cause more regurgitation than calcific degeneration as a result of leaflet retraction. Regurgitation may also follow aortic valve destruction in infective endocarditis.

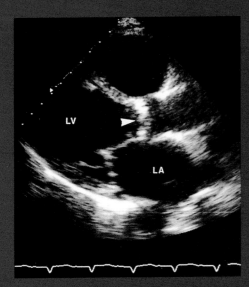

Fig 4.1 Calcific degenerative disease. Parasternal long-axis view (systole). The aortic cusps (arrow) should be open but have hardly moved from their closed position in diastole

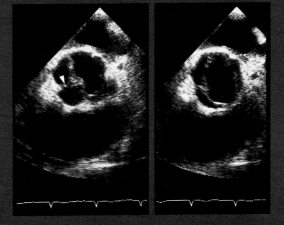

Fig 4.2 Bicuspid aortic valve, diagnosed by the presence of a median raphe (arrow) representing the unseparated cusp edges (transoesophageal view)

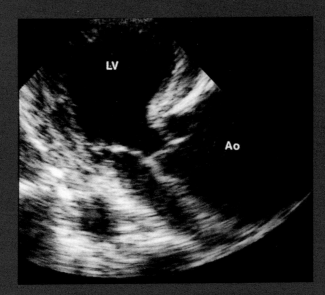

Fig 4.3 Aortic root dilatation (apical long-axis view) in a 75-year-old man with long-standing hypertension

Fig 4.4 Rheumatic mitral stenosis from the parasternal short-axis view. The leaflet tips are thickened and there is a highly echogenic spot (arrow) representing calcification or collagenous thickening where the medial commissure has become fused

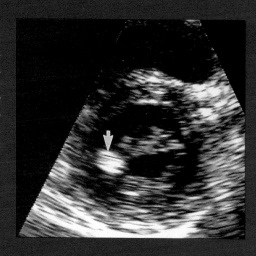

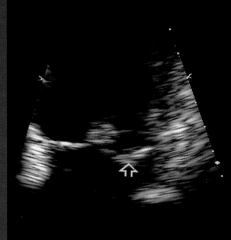

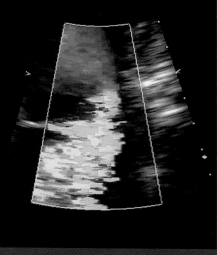

Fig 4.5 Mitral valve prolapse (apical four-chamber view). This view shows curvature of the posterior leaflet (arrow) above the plane of the annulus during systole in the left-hand panel with a broad jet or mitral regurgitation in the right-hand panel

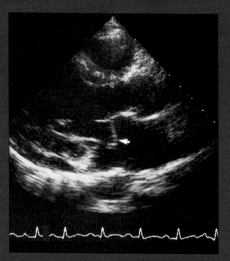

Fig 4.6 Mitral valve vegetation (arrowed) in a 25-year-old woman with fever and malaise

Mitral stenosis is almost exclusively rheumatic in origin (Figure 4.4). Mitral regurgitation is usually caused by left ventricular impairment leading to papillary muscle dysfunction or by mitral valve prolapse (Figure 4.5). Prolapse is defined by systolic movement of any part of either leaflet above the plane of the annulus in a long-axis view. Altogether at least 5% and up to 10% of all people have some degree of mitral prolapse. Some patients with prolapse have abnormal collagen (e.g. Marfan or Ehlers-Danlos syndromes), but others in whom there is minor 'technical' prolapse are effectively normal. Thus minor echocardiographic prolapse must not automatically be assumed to be the cause of non-specific symptoms. Antibiotic prophylaxis is usually recommended only if there is more than trivial mitral regurgitation in association with prolapse. However, this question is still debated periodically. Other causes of mitral regurgitation include rheumatic disease or endocarditis (Figure 4.6).

Murmurs as a result of intracardiac shunts in adults are most frequently caused by a secundum atrial septal defect (Figure 4.7). Ventricular septal defects are the most common congenital anomalies in children and, since a membranous defect frequently fails to close, these may also be found in adults. A patent ductus arteriosus is occasionally diagnosed for the first time in an adult.

Quantification of valve disease
Aortic stenosis

The mobility of the aortic cusps on the two-dimensional or M-mode scans gives an approximate guide to severity, but Doppler ultrasound gives a far more accurate assessment. Using continuous wave Doppler, the velocity of blood flow across the valve is directly related to the degree of stenosis, because a pressure difference (loosely called a 'gradient') across a stenotic valve must be accompanied by an increase in the velocity of blood flow. These parameters are approximately related by the simplified **Bernoulli equation**: $\Delta P = 4v^2$ (where ΔP is pressure difference in mmHg and v is the velocity in m/s) as long as the peak velocity is >3.0 m/s. For more mild aortic stenosis, this formula overestimates the pressure difference and no such estimate should usually be made. Mean pressure gradient is more accurate than peak gradient since it takes account of the whole rather than just the peak of the waveform. It is calculated automatically using online software by tracing round the waveform (Figure 4.8). The pressure difference estimated by Doppler echocardiography and cardiac catheterisation are related but different (Figure 4.9) and should not be compared directly (Rijsterborgh, 1987).

The pressure difference across the aortic valve is dependent on cardiac output. If flow is high as a result of anaemia or fever, the pressure difference

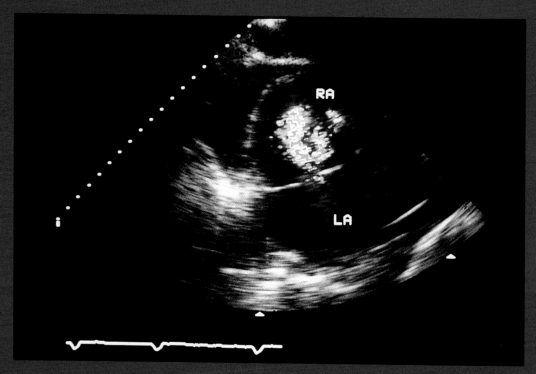

Fig 4.7 Secundum atrial septal defect (ASD). Subcostal view, clearly showing the origin of abnormal flow in the centre of the interatrial septum

Fig 4.8 Continuous wave recording from the apex in a patient with severe aortic stenosis. The signal has been planimetered giving an automated read-out of peak and mean pressure difference

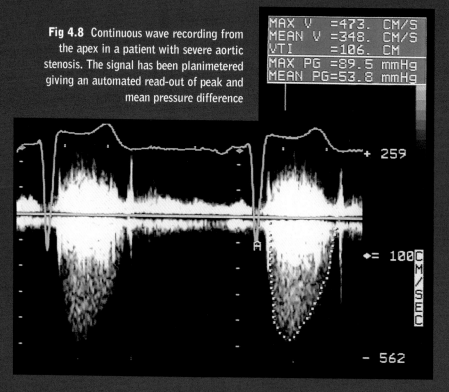

will be elevated. Conversely, in a patient with heart failure, the pressure difference may be low. In such patients it is necessary to correct for the effect of flow and this is most frequently done with the **continuity equation**. This is based on the law of conservation of mass (Figure 4.10) and allows an estimated 'effective' orifice area to be calculated (Table 4.2). This is a hydraulic area and is different from and usually smaller than the anatomic orifice area. The normal adult anatomic area is 2.5–3.5 cm².

Because of the square relationship between pressure and velocity, small errors in velocity measurement or small changes as a result of varying left ventricular function can lead to misclassification of grade. Thus a peak instantaneous velocity of 3.5 m/s equates with a moderate pressure difference of about 50 mmHg,

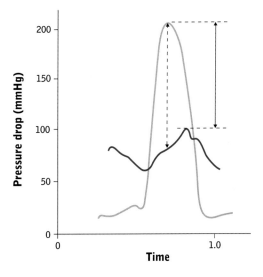

Fig 4.9 Doppler ultrasound measures the true peak instantaneous difference in pressure between the left ventricle and aorta (----). At catheterisation, it is usual to pull the catheter back across the aortic valve giving a 'pull-back' or 'peak-to-peak' gradient (——). The latter is not a true physiological pressure difference, as the peaks on the aortic and left ventricular pressure waveforms do not occur simultaneously

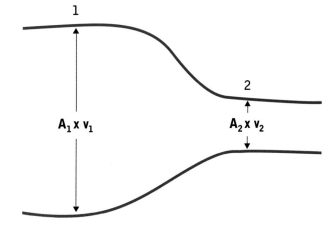

Fig 4.10 The principle of the continuity equation. The volume flow at point 1 (subaortic level) must be the same as at point 2 (aortic valve level). Assuming that the shape of the waveforms above and below the valve are similar, we can say that the cross-sectional area at 1 x velocity at 1 must equal area at 2 x velocity at 2. By rearrangement: Effective orifice area of the aortic valve is cross-sectional area of the subaortic region x subaortic peak velocity/ aortic peak velocity.

Subaortic velocity is recorded using pulsed Doppler with the sample in the left ventricular outflow tract; transaortic velocity is recorded using continuous wave Doppler

Table 4.2 Criteria for grading aortic stenosis

	Mild stenosis	Severe stenosis possible
Peak velocity (m/s)	<3.0	>4.0
Peak gradient (mmHg)	<35	>65
Mean gradient (mmHg)	<20	>40
Effective orifice area (cm^2)	>1.0	<0.75

N.B. Intermediate values may either represent moderate disease or, if left ventricular function is impaired, may represent severe disease. This distinction may require referral for a specialist opinion

whilst a velocity of 4.5 m/s equates with a severe pressure difference of 80 mmHg. Furthermore, the significance of a pressure difference varies between individuals depending largely on its effect on the left ventricle. Some patients with apparently moderate stenosis on haemodynamic criteria may become symptomatic and require operation, whilst others with high pressure differences may remain asymptomatic and be treated conservatively with relative safety.

Aortic regurgitation

Estimating the severity of regurgitation is more difficult than for aortic stenosis, and a balanced judgement must be made using a number of echocardiographic methods (Table 4.3) as well as the clinical examination. In general, Doppler is good for the diagnosis of severe aortic regurgiation but cannot reliably differentiate mild from moderate regurgitation. Severity of regurgitation is related to the area of failed valvar apposition (the 'regurgitant orifice'), the pressure difference across the valve in diastole, and various haemodynamic factors such as the heart rate and the ability of the left ventricle to expand during diastole. The size of the regurgitant orifice is related to the height of the jet on colour flow mapping (Figure 4.11). Severe regurgitation is likely if the jet occupies 60% or more of the full height of the left ventricular outflow tract. In severe aortic regurgitation, the pressure difference across the valve falls quickly and this shows as a steep deceleration slope on the continuous waveform (Figure 4.12). Normally, there is no diastolic flow reversal in the ascending aorta. In the presence of aortic regurgitation, there is flow reversal which lasts for longer during diastole and can be detected further down the aorta the more severe the regurgitation.

Table 4.3 Guideline criteria of severity in aortic regurgitation

Continuous wave pressure half-time	<400 ms
Continuous wave slope	>3.0 m/s^2
Colour flow height as proportion of LVOT height	>60%
Diastolic flow reversal at the aortic arch	present
Dilated volume loaded left ventricle	present

LVOT = left ventricular outflow tract

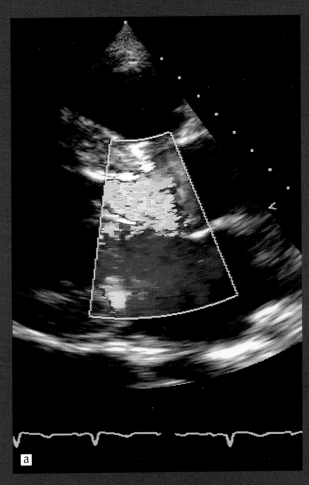

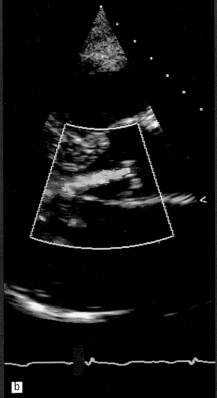

Fig 4.11 Aortic regurgitation on colour flow mapping. The size of the defect in the valve is related to the size of the base of the jet. A convenient measure is the height of the jet expressed as a percentage of the height of the subaortic outflow tract measured about 0.5 cm below the valve. Severe regurgitation is shown by a ratio greater than 60%. In (**a**) the jet fills the whole of the outflow tract; (**b**) shows mild regurgitation

Mitral stenosis

The mobility of the leaflet tips and the width of the colour flow map through the valve give approximate guides to severity, but the area of the orifice can be measured directly in the two-dimensional short-axis view. The orifice may be highly irregular and the reverberation from collagenous thickening or calcium deposits may make it impossible to trace the orifice accurately. The Doppler recording of flow across the valve gives a direct haemodynamic assessment (Figure 4.13). For historical reasons, the rate of fall of the velocity signal is usually expressed as the pressure half-time rather than the slope. The pressure half-time is the time taken for the peak gradient to fall by half. Because of the square relationship between pressure and velocity, the pressure half-time becomes the time for peak velocity to fall to $1/\sqrt{2}$ of its original value ($1/\sqrt{2} = 0.7$). Pressure half-time is inversely related to orifice area by an empirical orifice area formula:

$$\text{Mitral orifice area (cm}^2) = 220/\text{pressure half-time.}$$

This formula should not be applied if the pressure half-time is shorter than 150 ms, because in mild stenosis the half-time is significantly related to the diastolic behaviour of the left atrium and ventricle. Even in moderate or severe mitral stenosis, the pressure half-

time cannot produce a precise 'gold standard' orifice area. However, it is one of many useful guides to severity, which also include the speed of left ventricular filling and the pulmonary artery pressure.

The pulmonary artery pressure may be estimated from the transtricuspid pressure difference calculated from the tricuspid regurgitation jet using the Bernoulli equation added to an estimate of right atrial pressure. This is most accurately obtained from an assessment of the diameter of the inferior vena cava and its degree of collapse during inspiration.

The echocardiographer should then assess whether a valve is suitable for balloon valvotomy. This is a highly specialised judgement, which must be checked by transoesophageal echocardiography (TOE), but in general a valve is suitable if there is significant mitral stenosis with:

- Mobile and unthickened anterior leaflet base

- Little or no thickening of the chordae

- Tips not severely calcified

- No more than mild regurgitation

- No visible thrombus (Figure 4.14).

Table 4.4 Criteria of severity in mitral stenosis	
Measured orifice area (cm²)	< 1.0
Mean gradient (mmHg)	> 10
Pressure half-time (ms)	> 200
Estimated pulmonary artery pressure (mmHg)	> 35

Fig 4.12 The continuous wave signal in aortic regurgitation. In severe aortic regurgitation the pressure difference across the valve falls rapidly and the deceleration slope of the Doppler signal is correspondingly steep (arrows) (over 3 m/s²)

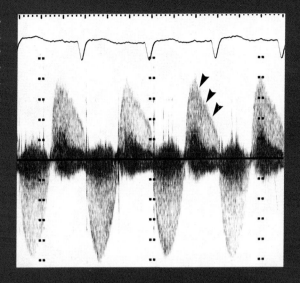

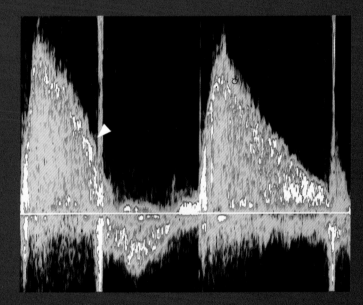

Fig 4.13 Mitral stenosis. On this continuous wave Doppler recording, velocities are raised throughout diastole, but are highly dependent on the length of the cycle. End-diastolic velocity is almost normal on the second complex but it is 1.6 m/s on the first (arrow)

Fig 4.14 Thrombus in the left atrial appendage (arrowed). Balloon mitral valvotomy was therefore cancelled and the patient referred for surgical valvotomy

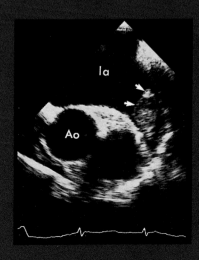

Mitral regurgitation

The regurgitant fraction depends mainly on the size of the regurgitant orifice, the length of time it remains open, the systolic pressure difference across the valve, and the distensibility of the left atrium. With continuous wave Doppler, the density of the signal, in comparison to forward flow, provides an approximate guide to severity (Figure 4.15). The greater the regurgitant fraction, the more red cells there are to scatter ultrasound and therefore the more dense the signal. The use of colour flow mapping to reflect the severity of mitral regurgitation is controversial. The area of the colour flow map is strongly dependent on the instrument settings and the type of echo machine used. However, a jet area $<4\,cm^2$ strongly suggests mild and an area $>8\,cm^2$ strongly suggests severe regurgitation (Spain, 1989) (Figure 4.16). There are also indirect measures of severity of regurgitation such as the activity of the left ventricle, the pulmonary artery pressure, and the behaviour of pulmonary venous flow pattern. Overall a balanced judgement must be made based on all these measures.

Shunts

The size of the shunt in the presence of an atrial or ventricular septal defect can be estimated from the ratio of the pulmonary to aortic stroke volume.

Table 4.5 Criteria of severity in mitral regurgitation

- Colour signal broad with prominent acceleration in the left ventricle
- Dense signal on continuous wave Doppler
- Systolic flow reversal in the pulmonary veins
- Volume overload of the left ventricle
- Raised pulmonary artery pressure

Which murmurs do not need echocardiography?

Benign systolic flow murmurs or the murmur of mild aortic valve thickening do not need echocardiography. These are frequent in high flow states, anaemia, fever, pregnancy, anxiety. They have the following characteristics:

- Short
- Soft or moderate in amplitude
- Ejection character
- Normal second heart sound
- May be louder on inspiration or lying.

Which patients should be referred to a cardiologist?

The following groups are the minimum that should be referred for specialist advice:

- Any symptomatic patient since the presence of symptoms is a criterion for surgery in all types of valve disease.

- Severe disease even in the absence of symptoms. Although surgery may not usually be performed in patients with severe aortic stenosis in the absence

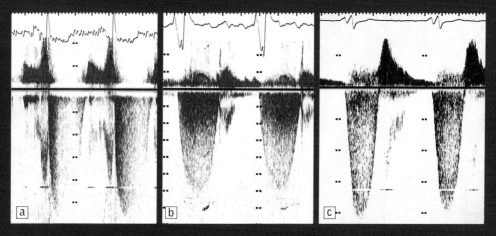

Fig 4.15 Mitral regurgitation continuous wave Doppler recording: **(a)** shows the low-intensity jet of mild regurgitation, **(b)** a medium jet, and **(c)** the dense jet of severe regurgitation

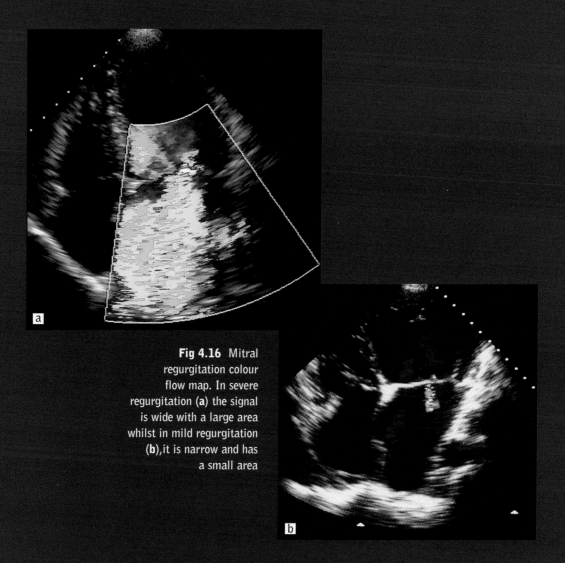

Fig 4.16 Mitral regurgitation colour flow map. In severe regurgitation **(a)** the signal is wide with a large area whilst in mild regurgitation **(b)**, it is narrow and has a small area

of symptoms there remains a small risk of sudden death and surgery may still be performed prophylactically. Similarly, in mitral stenosis where the left ventricle is protected by being downstream from the valve lesion, it is uncommon to operate in the absence of symptoms. However, the right ventricle may fail as a result of pulmonary hypertension and symptoms then diminish. The development of early right ventricular dysfunction on echocardiography is a warning sign arguing for prophylactic surgery.

- Moderate aortic or mitral regurgitation. The timing of surgery for patients with severe regurgitant lesions is often difficult. There is the danger of leaving this so late that irreversible left ventricular damage supervenes. Furthermore, because the assessment of regurgitation is less precise than for stenotic lesions, it is safer to refer even patients with apparently moderate disease.

- Any suggestion of impaired left ventricular systolic function. If the left ventricle is impaired, the severity of aortic stenosis may be under-estimated. Furthermore, a reduction in measures of left ventricular systolic function represents a criterion for operating in aortic stenosis and both aortic and mitral regurgitation.

References

Hall, R.J.C. and Julian, D.G. *Diseases of the Cardiac Valves*. Edinburgh: Churchill Livingstone, 1989

Lindroos, M., Kupari, M., Heikkilä, J. and Tilvis, R. Prevalence of aortic valve abnormalities in the elderly: an echocardiographic study of a random population sample. *JACC* 1993; **21**: 1220–5

Rijsterborgh, H. and Roelendt, J. Doppler assessment of aortic stenosis: Bernoulli revisited. *Ultrasound Med. Biol.* 1987; **13**: 241–8

Spain, M.G., Smith, M.D., Grayburn, P.A., Harlamert, E.A. and DeMaria, A.N. Quantitative assessment of mitral regurgitation by Doppler color flow imaging: angiographic and hemodynamic correlations. *JACC* 1989; **13**: 585–90

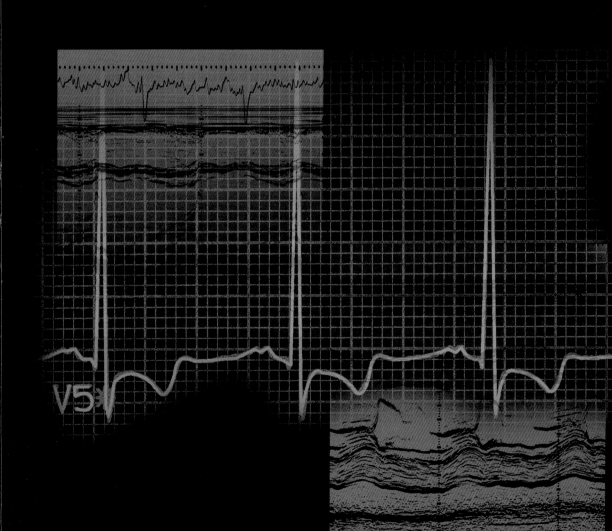

Left ventricular hypertrophy is an important risk factor for both myocardial infarction and sudden death, equivalent in impact to the presence of multivessel coronary disease (Liao, 1995). The relative risk for all cause mortality for every 50 g/m increase in mass is 1.5 in men and 2.0 in women (Levy, 1990). Left ventricular hypertrophy can therefore be used as an indication for treatment in patients with borderline hypertension. Patients with unequivocal hypertension need not have echocardiography since the decision to treat is based on the level of blood pressure alone. However, in young subjects, echocardiography should also be used to screen for coarctation. There is an argument for screening elderly patients with hypertension to look for aortic dilatation. Prophylactic surgery is indicated for an ascending aorta with a diameter >6.0 cm.

Electrocardiographic hypertrophy is diagnosed if QRS voltages are high or if the strain pattern is present. The voltage criterion (R in V5 plus S in V2 >45 mm) is non-specific since it may be seen in slim normal subjects (Figure 8.2). The strain pattern (Figure 5.1) consists of ST segment depression and T wave inversion in V5 and V6 sometimes associated with left-axis deviation. This is highly specific for left ventricular hypertrophy and is associated with a 7–9 times increased risk of heart failure in hypertensive patients. However, it is also insensitive. Overall, echocardiography is 5–10 times more sensitive at detecting left ventricular hypertrophy (Hammond, 1988). An electrocardiogram is therefore not a viable alternative to echocardiography.

Left ventricular hypertrophy is usually diagnosed by the presence of absolute septal thickening; this is an insensitive way of making the diagnosis (Figure 5.2). An estimate of left ventricular (LV) mass (in g) should be obtained, for example using the Devereux formula based on septal (S) and posterior (PW) wall thickness in diastole, as well as left ventricular diastolic diameter

Table 5.1 Indications for echocardiography	
Indication	**Goal**
Borderline hypertension	Left ventricular hypertrophy as evidence for treating or modifying therapy
Age <35 years	Aortic coarctation as a cause
In discussion	
Age >65 years	To detect aortic dilatation

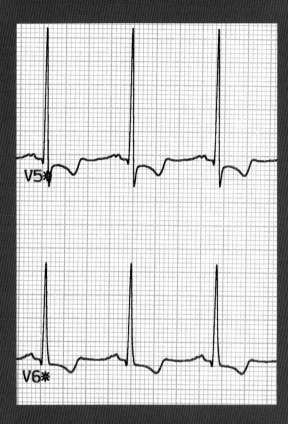

Fig 5.1 Electrocardiogram in left ventricular hypertrophy. There is ST segment depression and T wave inversion or left ventricular 'strain'

Fig 5.2 Echocardiogram in left ventricular hypertrophy. In (**a**) is an M-mode recording in a normal subject, in (**b**) from a patient with hypertension secondary to chronic renal failure

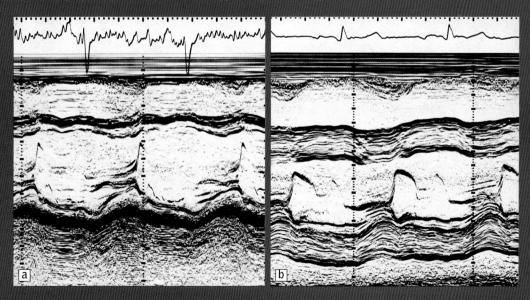

(LVDD) (Devereux, 1977):

$$LV\ mass = 1.04\,[(S + PW + LVDD)^3 - LVDD^3] - 13.6$$

This should then be indexed to body habitus, for example to body surface area. Well-accepted criteria for hypertrophy are left ventricular mass $> 134\,g/m^2$ in men and $> 110\,g/m^2$ in women (Hammond, 1988). The Devereux formula, based on M-mode echocardiography, should not be used if there are regional abnormalities of left ventricular function (e.g. myocardial infarction) or if the echocardiogram is of suboptimal quality. Two-dimensional methods of estimating left ventricular mass are more accurate (Reicheck, 1983), but not yet widely used.

References

Chambers, J.B. Left ventricular hypertrophy: an underappreciated coronary risk factor. *Br. Med. J.* 1995; **311**: 273–4

Devereux, R.B. and Reicheck, N.R. Echocardio-graphic determination of left ventricular mass in man: anatomic validation of the method. *Circulation* 1977; **55**: 613–8

Hammond, I.W., Devereux, R.B., Alderman, M.H., Lutas, E.M., Spitzer, M.C., Crowley, J.S. and Laragh, J.H. Prevalence and correlates of echocardiographic left ventricular hypertrophy among employed patients with uncomplicated hypertension. *JACC* 1988; **7**: 639–50

Liao, Y., Cooper R.S., McGee, D.L., Mensah, G.A., and Ghali, J.K. The relative effects of left ventricular hypertrophy, coronary artery disease and left ventricular dysfunction on survival among black adults. *JAMA* 1995; **273**: 1592–7

Levey, D., Garrison, R.J., Savage, D.D., Kannel, W.B. and Castelli, W.P. Prognostic implications of echocardiographically determined left ventricular mass in the Framington Heart Study. *N.Engl. J. Med.* 1990; **322**: 1561–6

Reicheck, N., Helak, J., Plappert, T., Sutton, M.St.J. and Weber, K.T. Anatomic validation of left ventricular mass estimates from clinical two-dimensional echocardiography: initial results. *Circulation* 1983; **67**: 348–52

Chapter 6

Atrial fibrillation

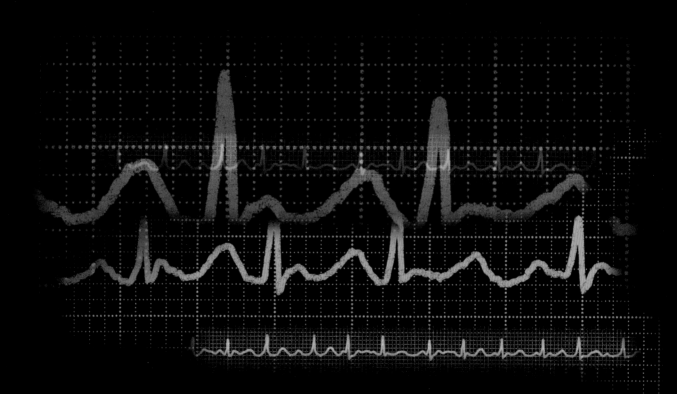

Atrial fibrillation (Figure 6.1) is not a complete diagnosis, and a number of underlying causes need to be looked for and excluded, including ischaemic heart disease, cardiomyopathy, hypertension, mitral valve disease, and thyrotoxicosis. Once done, and provided the patient is under 60 years of age, a diagnosis of lone atrial fibrillation can be made. For the purposes of treatment, there are effectively three categories of atrial fibrillation:

- rheumatic,
- non-rheumatic, and
- lone atrial fibrillation.

Lone atrial fibrillation is a benign condition which does not carry the risk of thromboembolism so that anticoagulation with warfarin is not required. The need for warfarin is clear in the presence of rheumatic disease. For non-rheumatic disease, there may be uncertainty over whether the benefit of anticoagulation outweighs the risk of bleeding. The benefit is a fall in the risk of stroke by 60% (Boston Trial, SPAF, 1992), while the risk of bleeding is variable (up to 5% per year, rising sharply beyond 80 years of age). Echocardiography can reasonably be used to aid this decision. There is some evidence that, with a normal echocardiogram, the risk of stroke is small, even with associated atrial fibrillation. However, this risk rises sharply if there is left atrial enlargement or left ventricular dysfunction (Table 6.1).

References

Boston Area Anticoagulation Trial for Atrial Fibrillation Investigators. The effect of low dose warfarin in the risk of stroke in patients with nonrheumatic atrial fibrillation. *N. Engl. J. Med.* 1990; **323**: 1505–11

Stroke Prevention in Atrial Fibrillation Study Group Investigators. Predictors of thromboembolism in atrial fibrillation. II. Echocardiographic features of patients at risk. *Ann. Intern. Med.* 1992; **116**: 6–12

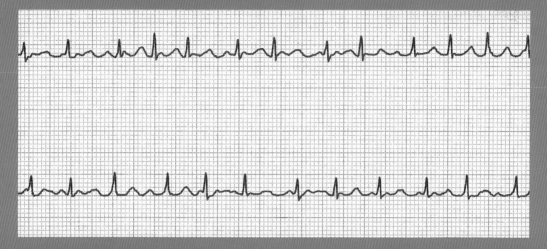

Fig 6.1 An electrocardiogram showing atrial fibrillation

Table 6.1 The annual risk of stroke rises if a patient has left atrial (LA) enlargement or left ventricular (LV) dysfunction

Findings	Annual risk (%)
Sinus rhythm (normal heart)	0.3
Lone atrial fibrillation (AF)	0.5
AF + normal echo	1.5
AF + LA > 2.5 cm/m²	8.8
AF + global LV dysfunction	12.6
AF + LA > 2.5 cm/m² and moderate LV dysfunction	20.00

Reference: Stroke Prevention in Atrial Fibrillation Study Group Investigators. Predictors of thromboembolism in atrial fibrillation. II Echocardiographic features of patients at risk. *Ann. Intern. Med.* 1992; **116**; 6–12   N.B. Left atrial area was used. This is not a widely-applied measure but is intuitively sensible

Chapter 7

Stroke and transient ischaemic attack

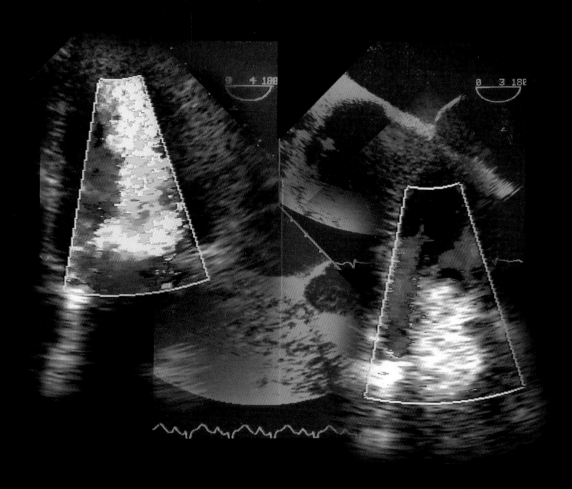

The single most useful investigation for transient ischaemic attacks other than in the vertebrobasilar artery territory is carotid duplex scanning since the finding of an internal carotid stenosis >70% by diameter is an indication for endarterectomy. By contrast, the diagnostic yield from transthoracic echocardiography is virtually zero in the absence of clinical or electrocardiographic (ECG) abnormalities, and should not be requested in their absence (Table 7.1). Within these appropriately narrow indications, the main purpose of echocardiography is to detect or confirm:

- a diagnosis known to be associated with a risk of thromboembolism, such as left ventricular dilatation or mitral stenosis.

- a direct source of emboli such as thrombus, myxoma or vegetation.

Of these, the presence of an underlying substrate for thromboembolism is the more important. Thus, the risk of thromboembolism is so high in the presence of mitral stenosis that it can be assumed to be the cause of cerebral infarction even in the absence of left atrial thrombus (which may be too small for detection or may already have embolised). The decision to anticoagulate with warfarin should never be made without a CT (computed tomographic) scan since haemorrhagic stroke can also occur in patients with atrial fibrillation.

However, occasionally, a direct source of emboli, usually a thrombus, is discovered (Figure 7.1). If there is a clinically obvious cause of stroke, echocardiography is still indicated since it may refine the diagnosis. An example is the detection of a ball thrombus (Figure 7.2) in a patient with mitral stenosis since this is an

Table 7.1 Indications for echocardiography in stroke or transient ischaemic attack

Transthoracic
Cerebral infarction on CT scanning and:

Abnormal ECG	Myocardial infarct
	Atrial fibrillation
	Nonspecific ST/T wave abnormalities
Abnormal signs	Murmur (other than short soft ejection systolic murmur)
	Endocarditis possible, e.g. vasculitis, high erythrocyte sedimentation rate

Transoesophageal
Cerebral infarction on CT scanning and normal or equivocal transthoracic study and:
- Likelihood of endocarditis
- Patients aged under 50 years (arbitrary)

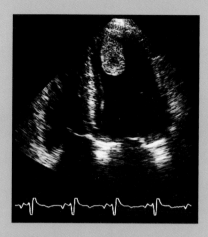

Fig 7.1 Left ventricular thrombus

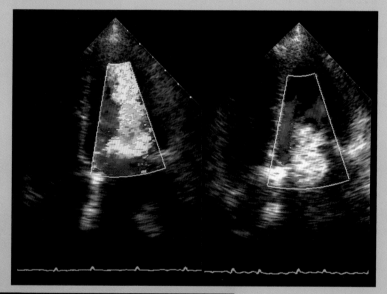

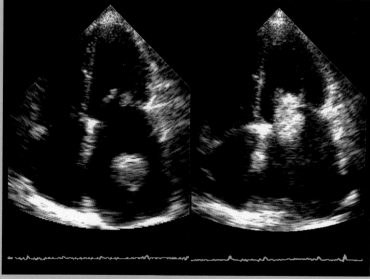

Fig 7.2 Ball thrombus in a patient with mitral stenosis. In systole, the thrombus lies towards the base of the greatly enlarged left atrium; in diastole it enters the mitral orifice virtually occluding forward flow

indication for urgent surgery.

In subjects aged under 50 years, it is generally accepted that a full study including transoesophageal echocardiography should be performed even in the absence of clinical abnormalities. This is mainly to look for rare treatable causes of stroke such as left atrial myxoma which occurs in 1% of such cases (Hart, 1983). Other abnormalities on transoesophageal echocardiography that may be relevant are left atrial spontaneous contrast (implying a higher than average risk of thrombo-embolism), patent foramen ovale (allowing the passage of venous thrombus from right to left heart) (Figure 7.3) and aortic atheroma.

References

Cerebral Embolism Task Force. Cardiogenic brain embolism. *Arch. Neurol.* 1989; **46**: 727–43

Chambers, J. B. The cardiac investigation of transient ischaemic attacks and stroke. In Jackson, G. (ed). *Difficult Concepts in Cardiology.* London: Martin Dunitz, 1994; pp157–81

Hart, R.G. and Miller, V.T. Cerebral infarction in young adults: a practical approach. *Stroke* 1983; **14**: 110–14

Schapiro, L.M., Westgate C.J., Shine, K. and Donaldson, R. Is cardiac ultrasound mandatory in all patients with systemic emboli? *Br. Med. J.* 1985; **291**: 786–7

Fig 7.3

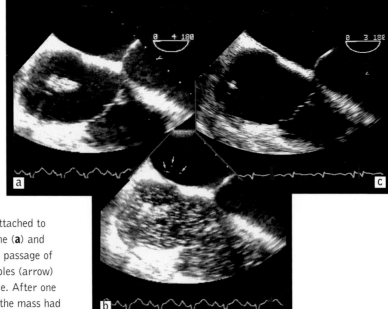

Transoesophageal echocardiography after stroke. The patient was a young woman with severe asthma controlled by regular injections of methyl prednisolone given via an indwelling subclavian line. She had a stroke followed by an embolism to the left leg. Echocardiography showed a thrombus attached to the right atrial part of the line (**a**) and contrast injection (**b**) showed passage of a small number of microbubbles (arrow) across a patent foramen ovale. After one week of intravenous heparin the mass had resolved (**c**)

Chapter 8

Screening

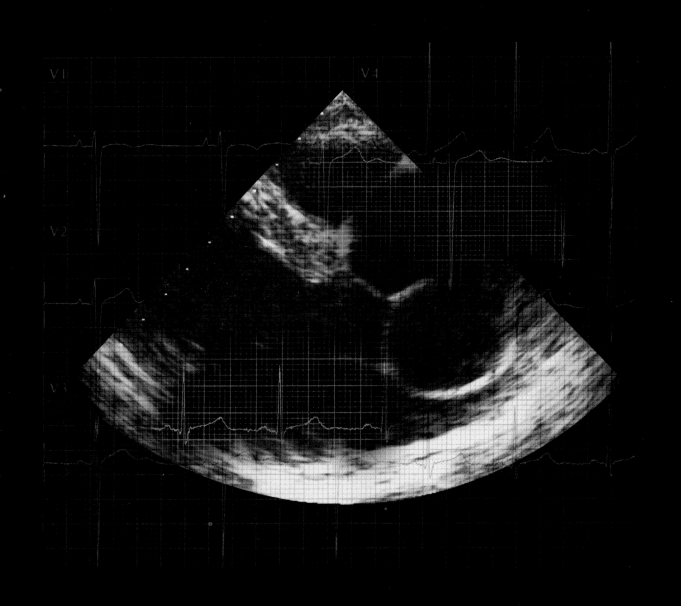

Echocardiography is indicated for:

- first-degree relatives of patients with hypertrophic cardiomyopathy

- suspected collagen abnormalities such as Marfan syndrome or Ehlers-Danlos syndrome.

Hypertrophic cardiomyopathy is familial in one-half of all cases and it is reasonable to offer screening to first-degree relatives of probands. There is no agreement about the age at which echocardiography should be performed in children. Many cardiologists study at 5 years, then every 5 years until the age of 20 years. However, the electrocardiogram alone may be a reliable screening tool and the presence of abnormal T waves used as an indication for echocardiography (Figure 8.1). Overzealous interpretation of the electrocardiogram should be carefully guarded against. Large voltages in a slim athletic individual are normal (Figure 8.2) and not an indication for echocardiography. Hypertrophic cardiomyopathy is rare with an incidence of only 0.4–2.5 per 100 000 population per year compared with up to 6.0 per 100 000 population for dilated cardiomyopathy.

In patients with suspected collagen abnormalities, echocardiography may show prolapse of the mitral and other valves, or dilatation of the aortic root (Figure 8.3) or other parts of the aorta.

There is a case for screening asymptomatic patients with a high chance of left ventricular dysfunction who might benefit from ACE inhibitors. This group includes patients after myocardial infarction or those with a high alcohol consumption. Another possible indication is hypertension since the finding of increased left ventricular mass might lead to a modification of therapy to include drugs known to induce left ventricular regression. However, there is insufficient evidence yet to justify screening these large groups of patients.

Regular echocardiographic follow-up is necessary for some groups of patients. There are no rigid rules, but a suggested plan is given in Table 8.1.

Table 8.1 Suggested minimum frequency of follow-up

- biological replacement valves – 5 years after implantation and every year thereafter (Chambers, 1994)
- severe aortic stenosis – 6 months
- moderate aortic stenosis – 12 months
- moderate aortic regurgitation – every 3–6 months
- hypertrophic cardiomyopathy – every 12 months
- dilated aortic root: initially every 6 months, if stable every 12 months.

Reference

Chambers, J. B., Fraser, A., Lawford, P., Nihoyannopoulos, P. and Simpson, I. Echocardiographic assessment of artificial heart valves: British Society of Echocardiography position paper. *Br. Heart J*. 1994; **71** (Suppl): 6–14

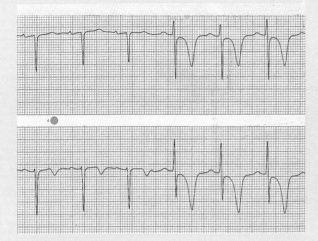

Fig 8.1 The electrocardiogram in hypertrophic cardiomyopathy. There are deeply inverted T waves across the chest leads

Fig 8.2 Normal electrocardiogram. This recording was made in a young, slim subject as a result of which he was referred on the suspicion of hypertrophic cardiomyopathy. Although the QRS voltages are a little high, they are within normal limits. Voltage criteria alone should not be an indication for echocardiography

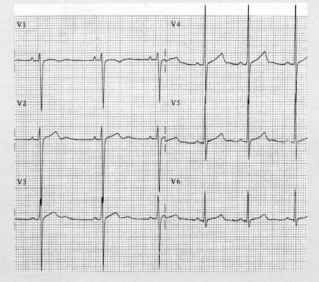

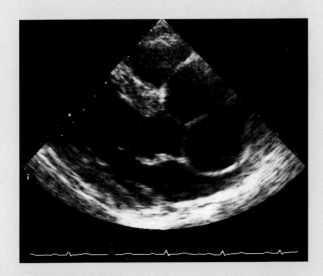

Fig 8.3 Dilatation of the sinuses of valsalva in a patient with Marfan syndrome